全国高等医药院校药学类实验教材

药物化学实验

（第二版）

主　编　孙铁民

编　者　（以姓氏笔画为序）

史济月　许佑君　孙铁民

沙　宇　赵　翔　赵冬梅

赵燕芳　贾　娴

中国医药科技出版社

内 容 提 要

本书为全国高等医药院校药学类实验教材之一。全书包括26个实验，覆盖药物化学实验的操作技术、药物合成的基本方法、药物结构修饰的基本方法。为适应教育国际化的要求，增加了英文对照内容，以便于学生在阅读英文文献、撰写英文论文时参考。

本书可作为高等医药院校药学、制药工程及相关专业实验教材使用，也可供医药院校教师及医药企业人员参考。

图书在版编目（CIP）数据

药物化学实验/孙铁民主编．—2版．—北京：中国医药科技出版社，2014.8
全国高等医药院校药学类实验教材
ISBN 978-7-5067-6935-8

Ⅰ.①药… Ⅱ.①孙… Ⅲ.①药物化学-化学实验-医学院校-教材 Ⅳ.①R914-33

中国版本图书馆CIP数据核字（2014）第171104号

美术编辑 陈君杞
版式设计 郭小平

出版 中国医药科技出版社
地址 北京市海淀区文慧园北路甲22号
邮编 100082
电话 发行：010-62227427 邮购：010-62236938
网址 www.cmstp.com
规格 787×1092mm 1/16
印张 10
字数 173千字
初版 2006年3月第1版
版次 2014年8月第2版
印次 2024年8月第9次印刷
印刷 北京印刷集团有限责任公司
经销 全国各地新华书店
书号 ISBN 978-7-5067-6935-8
定价 35.00元

全国高等医药院校药学类规划教材常务编委会

第二版前言

《药物化学实验》依据药物化学教学大纲的要求编定，目的是通过实验加深理解药物化学的基本理论和基本知识，掌握合成药物的基本方法；掌握对药物进行结构修饰的基本方法，了解拼合原理在药物化学中的应用；进一步巩固有机化学实验的操作技术及有关理论知识，培养学生理论联系实际、实事求是、严格认真的科学态度与良好的工作习惯。

在教学过程中，可针对不同的培养目标，选择相关实验。基本要求是课前作好预习，查阅有关文献和数据，了解实验的基本原理和方法，课后认真书写实验报告。

本实验教材源于教学实践经验，限于水平，难免有误，我们要在使用过程中不断总结修订，以便进一步修正提高。本次修订是在第一版教材基础上，根据药学教育发展需要，着眼于注重创新能力培养，全面提升学生的创新能力和思想的目的，增加了综合实验和开放实验内容，同时，增加了适合制药工程专业开设的药物化学实验和开放药物化学实验内容。各校可根据实际情况，选择适合本校情况的教学内容。欢迎批评指正。

编者

2014 年 5 月

contents

目录

实验一 阿司匹林（Aspirin）的合成

【目的要求】

1. 掌握酯化反应和重结晶的原理及基本操作。
2. 熟悉搅拌机的安装及使用方法。

【实验原理】

阿司匹林为解镇痛药，用于治疗伤风、感冒、头痛、发热、神经痛、关节痛及风湿病等。后来，又证明它具有抑制血小板凝聚的作用，其治疗范围又进一步扩大到预防血栓形成，治疗心血管疾病。

化学名：2-乙酰氧基苯甲酸

化学结构式：

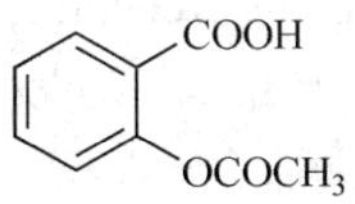

阿司匹林为白色针状或板状结晶，mp. 135℃ ~140℃，易溶乙醇，可溶于三氯甲烷、乙醚，微溶于水。

合成路线如下：

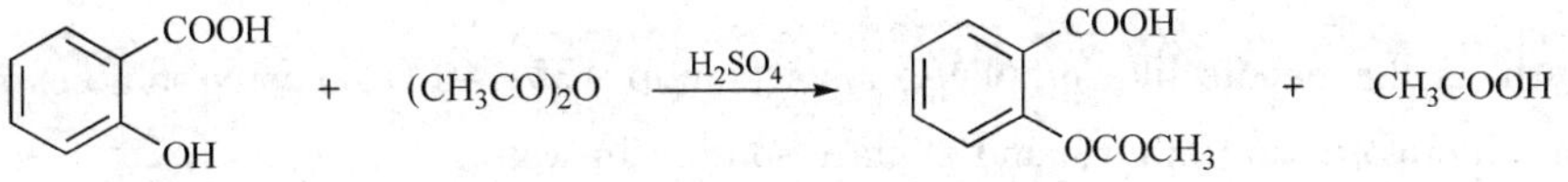

【实验方法】

（一）酯化

在装有搅拌棒及球形冷凝器的 100 ml 三颈瓶中，依次加入水杨酸 10 g，醋酐 14 ml，浓硫酸 5 滴。开动搅拌机，置油浴加热，待浴温升至 70℃时，维持在此温度反应 30 min。停止搅拌，稍冷，将反应液倾入 150 ml 冷水中，继续搅拌，至阿司匹林全部析出。抽滤，用少量稀乙醇洗涤，压干，得粗品。

（二）精制

将所得粗品置于附有球形冷凝器的 100 ml 圆底烧瓶中，加入 30 ml 乙醇，于水浴上加热至阿司匹林全部溶解，稍冷，加入活性炭回流脱色 10 min，趁热抽滤。将滤液慢慢倾入 75 ml 热水中，自然冷却至室温，析出白色结晶。待结晶析出完全后，抽滤，用少量稀乙醇洗涤，压干，置红外灯下干燥（干燥时温度不超过 60℃ 为宜），测熔点，计算收率。

（三）结构确证

1. 红外吸收光谱法、标准物 TLC 对照法。
2. 核磁共振光谱法。

【思考题】

1. 向反应液中加入少量浓硫酸的目的是什么？是否可以不加？为什么？
2. 本反应可能发生哪些副反应？产生哪些副产物？
3. 阿司匹林精制选择溶媒依据什么原理？为何滤液要自然冷却？

Experiment 1　Synthesis of Aspirin

Purpose

1. To master the principle and the basic operation of esterification and recrystallization.
2. To master the use and equipment of the agitator.

Mechanism

Aspirin is an antipyretic analgesic, which is used in the treatment of cold, headache, fever, neuralgia, arthralgia and rheumatic. Recently, it has been proved that it can restrain the agglomeration of blood platelet, and the scope of its treatment is enlarged to prevent the form of thrombus and cardiovascular disease.

Chemical name: 2-acetoxybenzoic acid, and chemical structure is as follow:

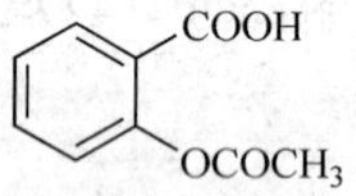

Aspirin is the needle-like or plate crystal, m. p. 135-140℃, easily soluble in ethanol, soluble in chloroform and ether, and slightly soluble in water.

The synthesis route is as follows:

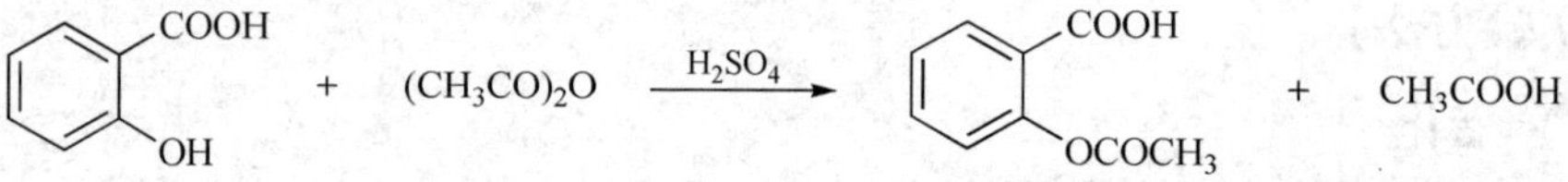

The experiment procedure

1. The esterification of salicylic acid

In a 100ml three-necked flask equipped with a reflux condenser and a stirrer bar, 10 g of salicylic acid, 14 ml of acetic anhydride and 5 drops of concentrated sulfuric acid are added and are heated to 70℃ with stirring for 30 minutes in an oil bath. Then the stirrer is stopped, and the reaction mixture is cooled for a while and is poured into 150 ml of cold water. It continued to stir until the crystal appeared. Then it is filtered, ished with a little dilute alcohol, and is pressed until it is dry. The crude product is obtained.

2. The refinement of aspirin

In a 100ml round bottom flask equipped with a spherical condenser, the crude product and 30 ml of ethanol are added. It is heated in the water bath until aspirin is completely dissolved. After cooled for a moment, the activated carbon is added and the mixture is discolored with reflux for 30 minutes. It is filtrated, poured into 75 ml of hot water and is cooled to room temperature naturally. Then all the crystal is precipitated. It is filtrated, ished with a little dilute ethanol, pressed until it is dry. The product is dried under the infrared lamp (the temperature should not be exceeded 60℃), and the melting point is measured and the yield is calculated.

3. Identification

1. Infrared absorption spectrometry, TLC confrontation method of the standard substance.

2. Nuclear magnetic resonance spectroscopy.

Questions

1. What is the purpose of the addition of a little concentrated sulfuric acid into the reaction mixture?

2. What kinds of side reaction will occur? What are the by-products?

3. What is the principle of solvent chosen in the refinement of aspirin? Why should the filtrate be cooled naturally?

实验二　扑炎痛（Benorylate）的合成

【目的要求】

1. 通过乙酰水杨酰氯的制备，了解氯化试剂的选择及操作中的注意事项。

2. 通过本实验了解拼合原理在化学结构修饰方面的应用。

3. 通过本实验了解 Schotten – Baumann 酯化反应原理。

【实验原理】

扑炎痛为一种新型解热镇痛抗炎药，是由阿司匹林和对乙酰氨基酚经拼合原理制成，它既保留了原药的解热镇痛功能，又减小了原药的毒副作用，并有协同作用。适用于急、慢性风湿性关节炎、风湿痛、感冒发热、头痛及神经痛等。

化学名：2-乙酰氧基苯甲酸-4-乙酰胺基苯酯

化学结构式：

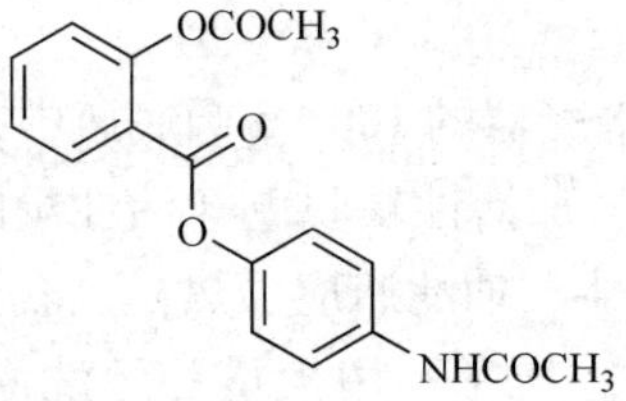

扑炎痛为白色结晶性粉末，无臭无味。mp. 174℃ ~178℃，不溶于水，微溶于乙醇，溶于三氯甲烷、丙酮。

合成路线如下：

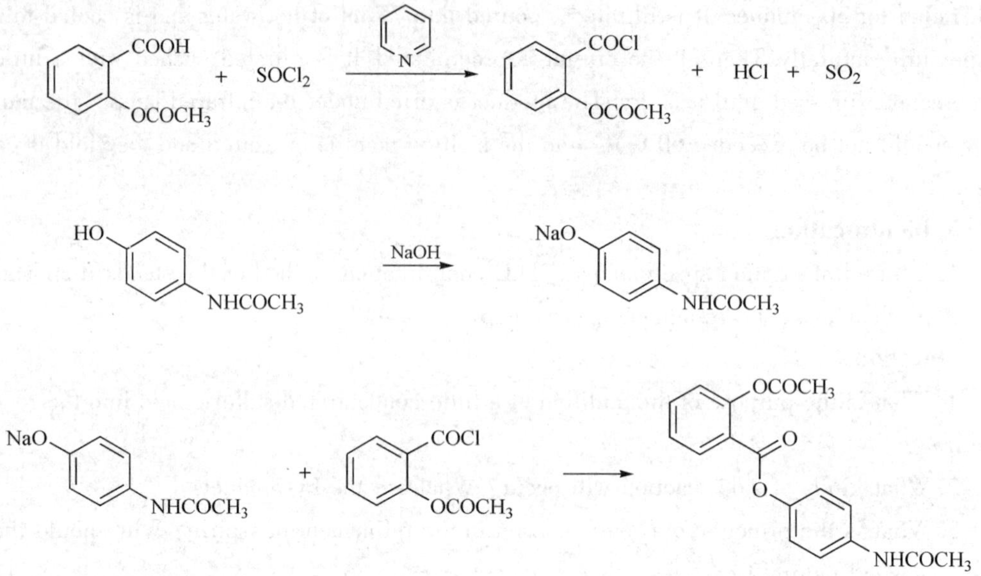

【实验方法】

（一）乙酰水杨酰氯的制备

在干燥的100 ml圆底烧瓶中，依次加入吡啶2滴，阿司匹林10 g，氯化亚砜5.5 ml，迅速按上球形冷凝器（顶端附有氯化钙干燥管，干燥管连有导气管，导气管另一端通到水池下水口）。置油浴上慢慢加热至70℃（约10～15 min），维持油浴温度在70℃±2℃反应70 min，冷却，加入无水丙酮10 ml，将反应液倾入干燥的100 ml滴液漏斗中，混匀，密闭备用。

（二）扑炎痛的制备

在装有搅拌棒及温度计的250 ml三颈瓶中，加入对乙酰氨基酚10 g，水50 ml。冰水浴冷至10℃左右，在搅拌下滴加氢氧化钠溶液（氢氧化钠3.6 g加20 ml水配成，用滴管滴加）。滴加完毕，在8℃～12℃之间，在强烈搅拌下，慢慢滴加上次实验制得的乙酰水杨酰氯丙酮溶液（在20 min左右滴完）。滴加完毕，调至pH≥10，控制温度在8℃～12℃之间继续搅拌反应60 min，抽滤，水洗至中性，得粗品，计算收率。

（三）精制

取粗品5 g置于装有球形冷凝器的100 ml圆底瓶中，加入10倍量（*W/V*）95%乙醇，在水浴上加热溶解。稍冷，加活性炭脱色（活性炭用量视粗品颜色而定），加热回流30 min，趁热抽滤（布氏漏斗、抽滤瓶应预热）。将滤液趁热转移至烧杯中，自然冷却，待结晶完全析出后，抽滤，压干；用少量乙醇洗涤2次（母液回收），压干，干燥，测熔点，计算收率。

（四）结构确证

1. 红外吸收光谱法、标准物TLC对照法。

2. 核磁共振光谱法。

［注释］

1. 二氯亚砜是将羧酸制备酰氯最常用的氯化试剂，不仅价格便宜而且沸点低，生成的副产物均为挥发性气体，故所得酰氯产品易于纯化。二氯亚砜遇水可分解为二氧化硫和氯化氢，因此所用仪器均需干燥；反应用阿司匹林需在60℃干燥4 h。吡啶作为催化剂，否则影响产品的质量。制得的酰氯不应久置。

2. 扑炎痛制备采用 Schotten – Baumann 方法酯化，即乙酰水杨酰氯与对乙酰氨基酚钠缩合酯化。由于对乙酰氨基酚酚羟基与苯环共轭，加之苯环上又有吸电子的乙酰胺基，因此酚羟基上电子云密度较低，亲核反应性较弱；成盐后酚羟基氧原子电子云密度增高，有利于亲核反应；此外，酚钠成酯，还可避免生成氯化氢，使生成的酯键水解。

【思考题】

1. 乙酰水杨酰氯的制备，操作上应注意哪些事项？

2. 扑炎痛的制备，为什么采用先制备对乙酰胺基酚钠，再与乙酰水杨酰氯进行酯化，而不直接酯化？

3. 通过本实验说明酯化反应在结构修饰上的意义。

Experiment 2 Synthesis of Benorylate

Purpose

1. Through the preparation of acetylsalicylic chloride to comprehend the choice of chlorination reagent and notes in the operation.

2. Through the experiment to comprehend the application of combination principles in chemical structure modification.

3. Through the experiment to master the theory of Schotten – Baumannesterification reaction.

Mechanism

Benorylate is a new antipretic, analgesic, counterplea medicine, and is synthesized by combination principles of aspirin and paracetamol. It retains the original antipyretic analgesic drug function, reduces the original drugs toxicities, and synergies. Applicable to the acute and chronic rheumatic arthritis, rheumatism and cold fever, headache and neuralgia, and so on.

Chemical name: 2-acetyl-*p*-phenyl ester acetamide; and chemical structure is as follow:

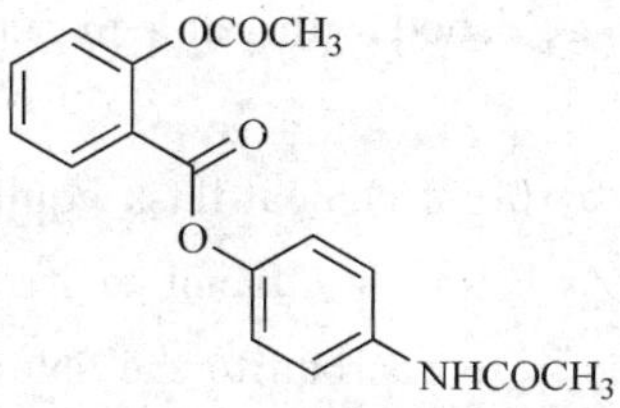

Benorylate is a white and crystal power, odorless and tasteless, m. p. 174 – 178℃, it is insoluble in water, slightly soluble in ethanol and dissolve in chloroform, acetone.

The synthesis route is below:

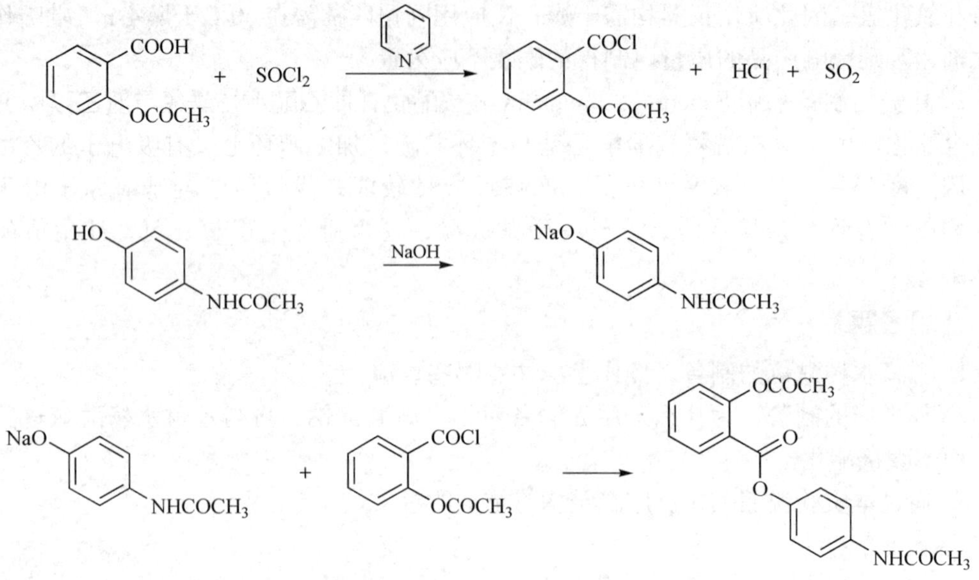

Experimental method

1. The preparation of acetylsalicylic chloride

In a dried 100ml conical flask, followed by adding two drops of pyridine, 10 g of aspirin, 5. 5 ml of thionyl chloride, quickly placed the spherical condenser on it(top equipped a drying tube with calcium chloride which is connected to airways, whose other end linked to pool). It is heated to 70℃ in the oil bath, (about 10-15min), and the temperature is kept in 70℃ ±2℃ for 70 min, cooled, and 10ml of anhydrous acetone are poured into the reaction solution, then the reaction solution is poured into a dried 100ml dropping funnel, standby.

2. The preparation of Benorylate

In a 250ml three neck flask equipped with a stirrer and a thermometer, place 10 g of paracetamol and 50 ml of water. It is cooled to 10℃ in ice water bath, and dropped sodium hydroxide solution(3. 6 g of sodium hydroxide is added to 20 ml of water) with a dropping tube. The solution of acetylsalicylic chloride and acetone is droped under vigorous stirring at 8 – 12℃ (about 20 min) . After Dropping, adjusted to pH ≥ 10, controlled the temperature at 8 – 12℃ for 60 minutes, filtering, ished with water to neutral, the yield is calculated.

3. Refinement

Place 5 g of crude product to a 100ml conical flask equipped with a spherical condenser, and add 10 times the volume (*W/V*) 95 % ethanol to it, heated to dissolve it in a water bath. Cool the solution, and add activated carbon to the soluntion (depending on crude color to determine the amount of activated carbon), reflux for 30 min and filtered (the Brinell funnel and bottles should be preheated). Filtrate will be transferred to the beaker, naturally cooled. After crystallization precipitates completely, filtered, pressed until it is dry; ished twice with a small amount of ethanol (from iste liquid), pressed until it is dry. The melting point is measured and the yield is calculated.

4. Structure Elucidation

(1) IR absorption spectroscopy, TLC standard material control law.

(2) NMR spectroscopy.

Notes

1. Thionyl chloride is a most commonly chlorination reagent used in preparation of chloride, it is nøt only cheap but also has low boiling point, by-products are volatile gases, easily obtained purified chloride products. Thionyl chloride can be decomposed into sulfur dioxide and hydrogen chloride in the water, so used equipments require drying; Aspirin should be dried at 60℃ for 4 h. The amount of pyridine should not be too large as a catalyst, otherwise it will affect the quality of products. The products should not be retained too long.

2. Benorylate is prepared by esterification method of Schotten-Baumann, that is, acetylsalicylic chloride condensates, and esterificates with paracetamol sodium. Because phenolic hydroxyl of paracetamol conjugates with the benzene ring, in addition to the electrophilic-acetyl amino in the benzene ring, phenolic hydroxyl is on the low density of the electron cloud, the pro-nuclear reaction is weaker; after salting, electronic cloud density of oxygen atom in phenolic hydroxyl increases, favorable to the pro – nuclear reaction. In addition, If phenol sodium is carbonated, it can prevent the formation of hydrogen chloride which results in ester hydrolysis.

Questions

1. During the preparation of acetylsalicylic chloride, which operations should be paid attention to?

2. In benorylate preparation, why is acetyl amino phenol sodium prepared firstly, then esterificated with acetylsalicylic chloride, instead of direct esterification?

3. To explain the significance of esterification reactions in the structural modification through this experiment.

实验三　水杨酰苯胺（Salicylanilide）的合成

【目的要求】

1. 了解对药物结构的修饰方法。
2. 掌握酚酯化和酰胺化的反应原理。

【实验原理】

水杨酰苯胺为水杨酸类解热镇痛药，用于发热、头痛、神经痛、关节痛及活动性风湿症，作用较阿司匹林强，副作用小。

化学名：2-羟基苯甲酰苯胺

化学结构式：

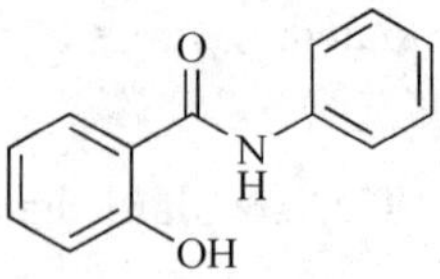

水杨酰苯胺为白色结晶性粉末，几乎无臭，微溶于冷水，略溶于乙醚、三氯甲烷、丙二醇，易溶于碱性溶液。mp. 135. 8℃ ~136. 2℃。

合成路线如下：

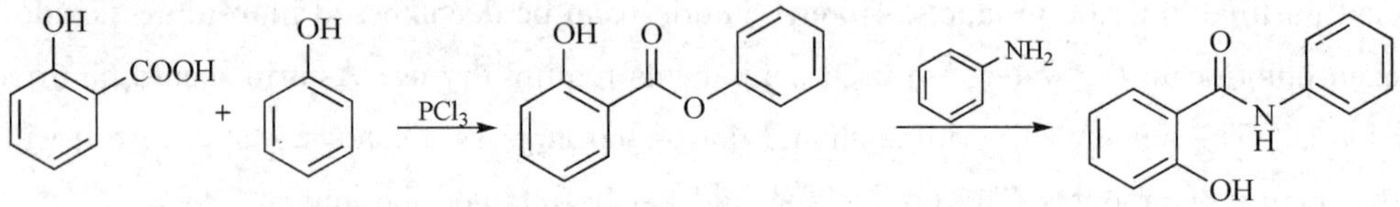

【实验方法】

（一）水杨酸苯酯的制备

在干燥的 100 ml 三颈瓶上安装搅拌器、温度计和球形冷凝器，依次加入苯酚 5 g，水杨酸 7 g，油浴加热使熔融，控制油浴温度在 140℃ ±2℃之间，通过滴液漏斗缓缓加入三氯化磷 2 ml，此时有氯化氢气体产生。在冷凝器上端接一排气管，尾管甩进水槽中，三氯化磷加毕，维持油浴温度在 140℃ ±2℃之间，反应 2 h，趁热搅拌下倾入 50 ml水（50℃）中，于冰水浴中不断搅拌，直至固化，过滤、水洗，得粗品。

（二）水杨酰苯胺的制备

将上步制得的水杨酸苯酯，投入 25 ml 圆底烧瓶，油浴加热至 120℃，使熔融，不时摇动圆底烧瓶，并在此温度维持 5 min 左右，然后按 1 g 水杨酸苯酯加 0. 45 ml 苯胺的比例，加入苯胺，安装回流冷凝器，加热至 160℃ ±5℃，反应 2 h，温度稍降后，趁热倾入 30 ml 85% 乙醇中，置冰水浴中搅拌，直至结晶析出，过滤，用 85% 乙醇洗 2 次，干燥，得粗品。

（三）精制

取粗品，投入附有回流冷凝器的圆底烧瓶中，加 4 倍量的（*W/V*）的 95% 乙醇，在 60℃水浴中，使之溶解，加少量活性炭及 EDTA 脱色 10 min，趁热过滤，冷却、过滤。用少量乙醇洗 2 次（母液回收）。干燥得本品。测熔点，计算收率。

（四）结构确证

1. 红外吸收光谱法、标准物 TLC 对照法。

2. 核磁共振光谱法。

[注释]

1. 本实验采用先合成水杨酸苯酯，然后再将苯胺酰化，而不是直接用水杨酸酰化。这是因为，氨基中的氮原子的亲核能力较羟基的氧原子强，一般可用羧酸或羧酸酯为酰化剂，而酯基中则以苯酯最活泼，且避免了羧酸与氨基物成盐的问题，因此羧酸酯类作为酰化剂常被应用。

2. 产品精制需加少量 EDTA，因为酚羟基易受金属离子催化氧化，使产品带有颜色。加入 EDTA 的目的是络合掉金属离子，防止产品氧化着色。

【思考题】

1. 水杨酰苯胺的合成，可否用水杨酸直接酯化？
2. 根据所学知识解释羧酸酯为酰化试剂时，为何苯酯的最为活泼？
3. 产品精制时，为什么要在 60℃使之溶解？脱色时为什么要加入少量 EDTA？

Experiment 3　Synthesis of Salicylanilide

Purpose

1. To understand the modification method of the structure of medicines.
2. To master the mechanism of the esterification and amidation of phenol.

Mechanism

Salicylanilide is an antipyretic analgesic of salicylic acid, which is used to treat with the febrile, headache, neuralgia, arthralgia and beriberoid disease. Its effect is stronger than Aspirin and the side effect is weaker.

Chemical name : *orth*-hydroxy benzoyl aniline; and the chemical structure is below:

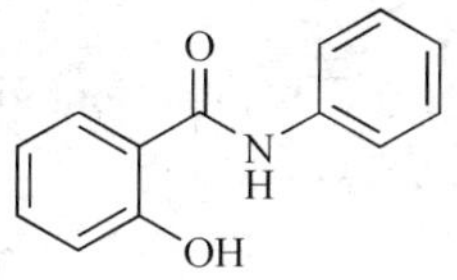

Salicyclanilide is a white crystallinity powder and almost odorless, which is slightly soluble in cold water, sparingly soluble in ether, chloroform, propylene glycol, and easily dissolved in alkaline solution. mp. 135. 8-136. 2℃.

The route of synthesis is below:

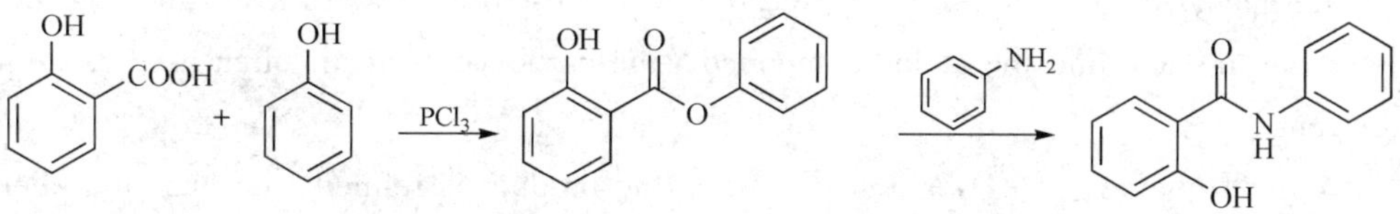

Procedure

1. Preparation of phenol salicylate

To a 100ml dried three – necked bottle equipped with an agitator, a thermometer and a reflux condenser, 5g of phenol and 7g of salicylic acid are added and are heated in an oil bath at 140 ± 2℃. 2ml of phosphorus trichloride is added slowly through a dropping funnel. The generated gas, chloride hydrogen, is introduced into the sink through a pipe which is equipped at the top of the condenser. The temperature of the oil bath is kept at 140 ±2℃. The mixture is reacted for 2h, then poured into 50ml of water (50℃) and is stirred in the ice water bath until solidified. After it is filtered and ished with water, the crude product is obtained.

2. Preparation of the salminidol

The product above is placed in a 25ml round – bottom flask and is heated to 120℃ in an oil bath. The flask should be shaked occasionally. It is kept at the temperature for 5 min. Then the aniline is added with the proportion (0. 45 ml of aniline per 1 g of phenol salicylate). The reflux condenser is equipped. The mixture is heated to 160℃ ±5℃ and is reacted for 2h. It is cooled for a moment and 30 ml of 85% ethanol is poured into. It is stirred in the ice water bath until the crystal is separated. The product is filtered and ished with 85% ethanol for two times. The crude product is obtained after dried.

3. Refinement

The crude product is placed in a round – bottom flask equipped with the reflux condenser, and 4 fold(*W/V*) of 95% ethanol is added. The mixture is dissolved in the 60℃ water bath. A small quantity of active carbon and EDTA are added and the mixture is decolored for 10min. It is filtered by hot, cooled filterate. It is ished with a small quantity of ethanol for two times (the mother liquid is recovered). The product is dried. Measure the melting point and calculate the yield.

4. Identification

① Infrared absorption spectrometry, TLC confrontation method of the standard substance.

② Nuclear magnetic resonance spectroscopy.

Notes

1. In this experiment, the phenol salicylate is synthesized in the first place and the aniline is acylated later, else not acylated the salicylic acid directly. Generally the carboxylic acid and the carboxylic ester are used as the acylating agent, because the nucleophilic competence of the nitrogen atom in the amino group is stronger than that of the oxygen atom in the hydroxyl group. The phenyl-ester is the most active group in the esterfunction. To avoid forming the salt of the carboxylic acid and the amino compound, the carboxylic ester is often used as the acylating agent.

2. A small quantity of EDTA is added when the product is refined, because the phenolic hydroxyl group is catalyticly oxidated by the metal ion easily which induced the product to have some color. The purpose of adding EDTA is to complex the metal ion in order to prevent the product from oxidation and coloration.

Questions

1. Whether can the salicylic acid be esterified directly when the salminidol is synthesized?

2. When the carboxylic ester used as the acylating agent, the phenyl – ester is the most active. To explain the reason.

3. Why should the product be dissolved at 60℃ when refined? Why is a small quantity of EDTA added when decoloration?

实验四 阿司匹林铝（Aluminum Acetylicylate）的合成

【目的要求】

1. 了解药物结构修饰方法。
2. 掌握减压蒸馏的基本操作。

【实验原理】

阿司匹林临床应用极为广泛，但在大剂量口服时，对胃黏膜有刺激作用，甚至引起胃出血。为克服这一缺点，常做成盐、酯和酰胺。阿司匹林铝即是其中之一，它的疗效和阿司匹林相近，但对胃黏膜刺激性较小。

化学名：羟基双（乙酰水杨酸）铝

化学结构式：

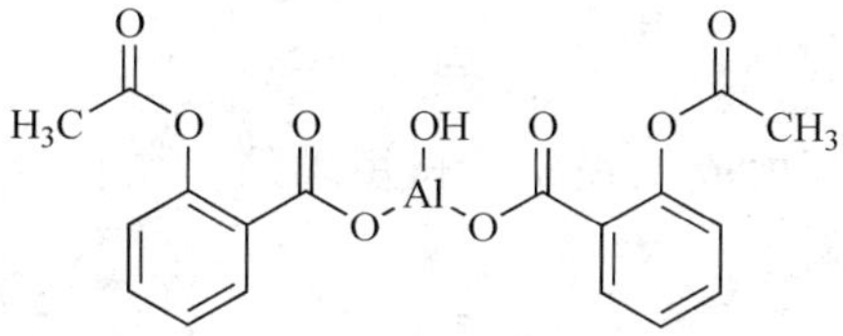

阿司匹林铝为白色或类白色粉末，几乎不溶于水和有机溶剂，溶于氢氧化碱或碳酸碱水溶液中，同时分解。

合成路线如下：

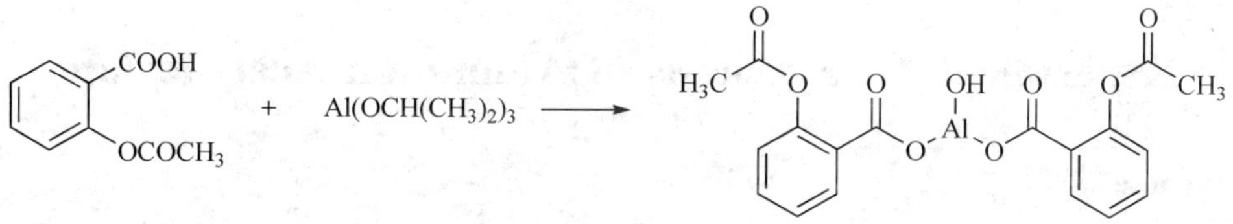

【实验方法】

（一）异丙醇铝的制备

称取1.8 g铝片，剪细，置100 ml圆底烧瓶中，加入少许二氯化汞，异丙醇20 ml，装好回流冷凝器及干燥管，油浴加热至沸腾，从冷凝器上口加入四氯化碳2滴，维持油浴温度120℃左右，加热回流至铝片全部消失（约1.5～2 h），溶液呈黑灰色，改为减压蒸馏装置。水泵减压回收异丙醇，然后用油泵减压蒸出异丙醇铝（142℃～150℃/25 mmHg）。得透明油状物或白色蜡状物。计算收率。

（二）阿司匹林羟基铝的制备

称取异丙醇铝6.8 g，置100 ml三颈瓶中，加异丙醇14 ml，开动搅拌，于油浴中加热至45℃（内温），溶液呈乳白色混浊，搅拌下加入阿司匹林12 g，几分钟后溶液呈透明，控制反应温度55℃～57℃（不要超过60℃），搅拌30 min，冷却至30℃，搅拌下加入40 ml异丙醇和水的混合液（37 ml异丙醇和3 ml水），形成大量白色沉淀，再于30℃下搅拌30 min，抽滤，用异丙醇10 ml洗一次，干燥得白色粉末状产品。计算收率。

（三）结构确证

1. 红外吸收光谱法、标准物TLC对照法。

2. 核磁共振光谱法。

［注释］

1. 加入的二氯化汞的量以直径为1 mm大小的颗粒为宜，直径大导致反应速度慢。

2. 加入异丙醇和水的混合液进行水解反应时，由于阿司匹林分子中的乙酰氧基和铝原子呈络合状态，故在本实验条件下，乙酰基不会水解下来。

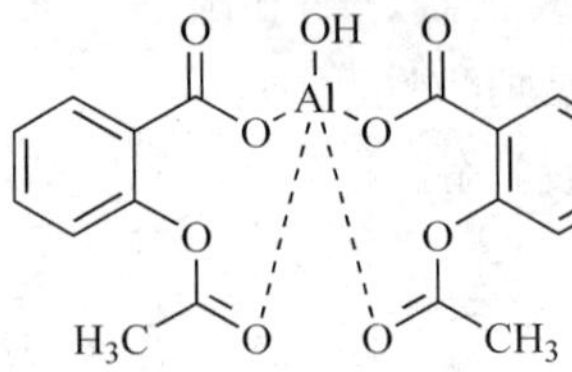

3. 铝片应剪成细丝，要剪成细长状，长短均匀，如有少量铝丝不溶，也应水泵减压蒸出异丙醇，不影响产量。

【思考题】

1. 试述减压蒸馏的操作要点。

2. 试述常用药物成盐方法及意义。

3. 试解释为何阿司匹林铝比阿司匹林副作用小。

Experiment 4　Synthesis of Aluminum Acetylicylate

Purpose

1. To understand the modification method of a drug' s structure.

2. To master the basic operation of vacuum distillation

Mechanism

Aspirin is extensively used in clinical application, but it will bring the stimulation to the gastric mucous membrane and even produce the gastrorrhagia when large dose for taken orally. So it is often made into the salt, ester or amide of aspirin to overcome this shortcoming. Aluminum Acetylicylate is one of them, and the effect is similar to the Aspirin, but the stimulation to the gastric mucous membrane is tiny.

Chemical name: hydroxyl di(acetyl salicylic acid)aluminum; and the chemical structure is below:

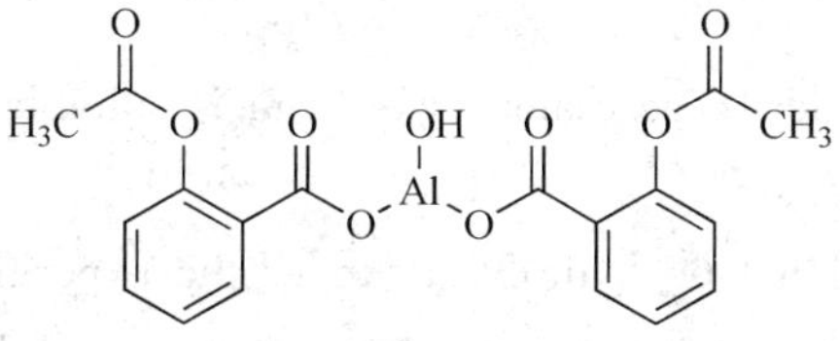

Aluminum Acetylicylate is a white or off-white powder, which is hardly solved in water and organic solvent but dissolved in the aqueous solution of the alkali hydroxide and the carbonate alkali decomposed at the same time.

The route of synthesis is below:

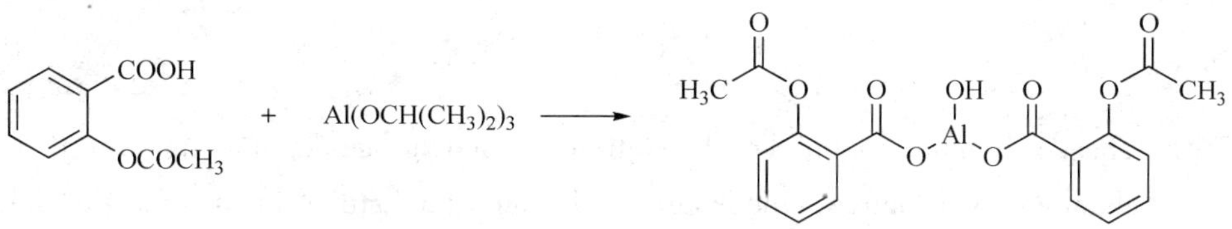

Procedure

1. Preparation of Aluminum isopropanol

1. 8 g of sheet aluminum is sliced thin and placed into a 100 ml flask, then a small quantity of mercury bichloride and 20 ml of isopropanol are added. The reflux condenser and drying cube are equipped. It is heated to boil in an oil bath. Then 2 drops of carbon tetrachloride are added from the condenser. The temperature of the oil bath is kept about 120℃. It is refluxed till the sheet aluminum is disappeared (about 1. 5-2 h). At that time the solution is charcoal grey. Install the vacuum distillation apparatus, and the isopropanol is collected through vacuum distillation with the water pump. And the aluminum isopropanol is collected through vacuum distillation with the oil pump (142-150℃/25 mmHg), which is transparent oil or white lardaceous material. The yield is calculated.

2. Preparation of Aluminum Acetylicylate

6. 8 g of aluminum isopropanol and 14 ml of isopropanol are placed in a 100 ml three – necked bottle. It is stirred and heated to 45℃ (intra temperature) in an oil bath. The solution is the ivory turbidity. 12g of Aspirin is added while stirred and the mixture is transparent for several minutes later. It is stirred for 30 min at 55-57℃ (do not exceed 60℃). It is cooled to 30℃ and added 40 ml mixture solution of isopropanol and water (composed of 37 ml of isopropanol and 3 ml of water). A lot of white precipitate is formed. It is stirred for 30 min at 30℃. Then be sucking filtrated and ished with 10 ml of isopropanol and dried. The white powder product is obtained. The yield is calculated.

3. Identification

(1) Infrared absorption spectrometry, TLC confrontation method of the standard substance.

(2) Nuclear magnetic resonance spectroscopy.

Notes

1. The mercury bichloride whose diameter is 1mm is suitable, because it will slow down the reaction with bigger particle.

2. The acetyl group will not be hydrolyzed under the experiment condition when the hydrolysis is carried out by adding the mixture solution of isopropanol and water, because the acetyl group and the aluminum are in complex state.

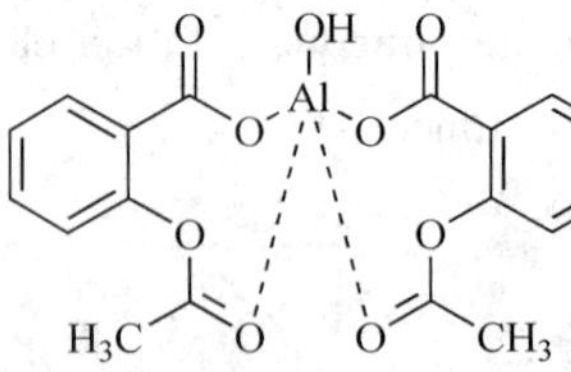

3. The sheet aluminum should be sliced thin, which is slender and uniform. If a small quantity of aluminum is insoluble, the isopropanol should be distilled in vacuum with the water pump and the yield will not be affected.

Questions

1. Try to state the main manipulative points of the vacuum distillation.

2. Try to state the normal methods and significance of salification of medicine.

3. The side effect of Aluminum Acetylicylate is weaker than that of Aspirin, try to state the reason.

实验五　苯妥英锌（Phenytoin-Zn）的合成

【目的要求】

1. 学习二苯羟乙酸重排反应机理。

2. 掌握用三氯化铁氧化的实验方法。

【实验原理】

苯妥英锌可作为抗癫痫药，用于治疗癫痫大发作，也可用于三叉神经痛。

化学名：5,5-二苯基乙内酰脲锌。

化学结构式：

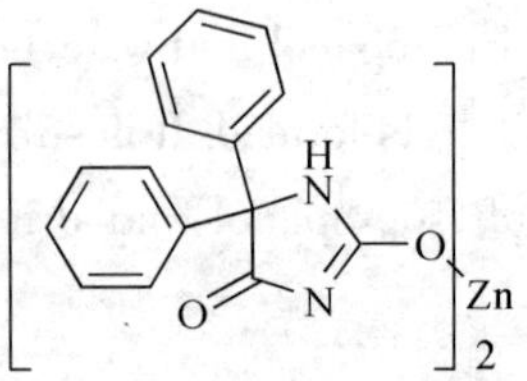

苯妥英锌为白色粉末，mp. 222℃～227℃（分解），微溶于水，不溶于乙醇、三氯甲烷、乙醚。

合成路线如下：

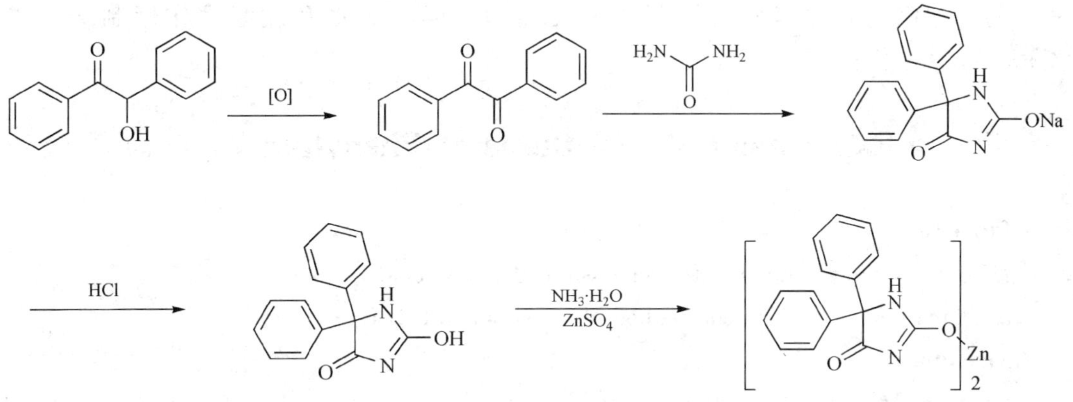

【实验方法】

（一）联苯甲酰的制备

在装有球形冷凝器的 250 ml 圆底烧瓶中，依次加入 $FeCl_3 \cdot 6H_2O$ 14 g，冰醋酸 15 ml，水 6 ml 及沸石一粒，在石棉网上直火加热沸腾 5 min。稍冷，加入安息香 2.5 g 及沸石一粒，加热回流 50 min。稍冷，加水 50 ml 及沸石一粒，再加热至沸腾后，将反应液倾入 250 ml 烧杯中，搅拌，放冷，析出黄色固体，抽滤。结晶用少量水洗，干燥，得粗品，测熔点，mp. 88℃～90℃，计算收率。

（二）苯妥英的制备

在装有球形冷凝器的 100 ml 圆底烧瓶中，依次加入联苯甲酰 2 g，尿素 0.7 g，20% 氢氧化钠 6 ml，50% 乙醇 10 ml 及沸石一粒，直火加热，回流反应 30 min，然后加入沸水 60 ml，活性炭 0.3 g，煮沸脱色 10 min，放冷过滤。滤液用 10 % 盐酸调 pH 6，析出结晶，抽滤。结晶用少量水洗，干燥，得粗品，计算收率。

（三）苯妥英锌的制备

将苯妥英 0.5 g 置于 50 ml 烧杯中，加入氨水（15 ml $NH_3 \cdot H_2O$ + 10 ml H_2O），尽量使苯妥英溶解，如有不溶物抽滤除去。另取 0.3 g $ZnSO_4 \cdot 7H_2O$ 加 3 ml 水溶解，然后加到苯妥英铵水溶液中，析出白色沉淀，抽滤，结晶用少量水洗，干燥，得苯妥英锌，称重，测分解点，计算收率。

（四）结构确证

1. 红外吸收光谱法、标准物 TLC 对照法。
2. 核磁共振光谱法。

［注释］

1. 制备联苯甲酰时，直火加热至中沸，通过测其熔点控制质量。
2. 苯妥英锌的分解点较高，测时应注意观察。

【思考题】

1. 安息香氧化制备联苯甲酰时，还可以用哪些氧化剂？酸性高锰酸钾可不可以？
2. 试述二苯羟乙酸重排的反应机理。

3. 为何不利用第二步反应中已生成的苯妥英钠，直接同硫酸锌反应制备苯妥英锌，而是把已生成的苯妥英钠制成苯妥英后，再与氨水和硫酸锌作用制备苯妥英锌？

Experiment 5　Synthesis of Phenytoin Zinc

Purpose

1. To study the rearrangment mechanism of benzilic acid

2. To master the experiment mathod of oxidation with $FeCl_3$.

Mechanism

Phenytoin Zinc can be used as an antiepileptic for the treatment of grand mal epilepsy or trifacial neuralgia.

Chemcal name：5,5-diphenylhydantoin Zinc；and the chemcal structure is below：

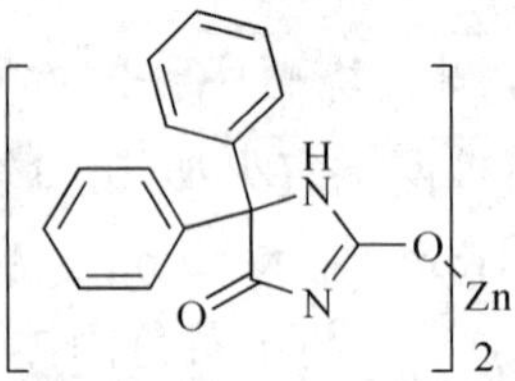

Phenytoin Zinc is a white powder，mp. 222-227℃（dec.），which is slightly soluble in water，but dissoluble in ethanol，chloroform and ether.

The synthesis route is below：

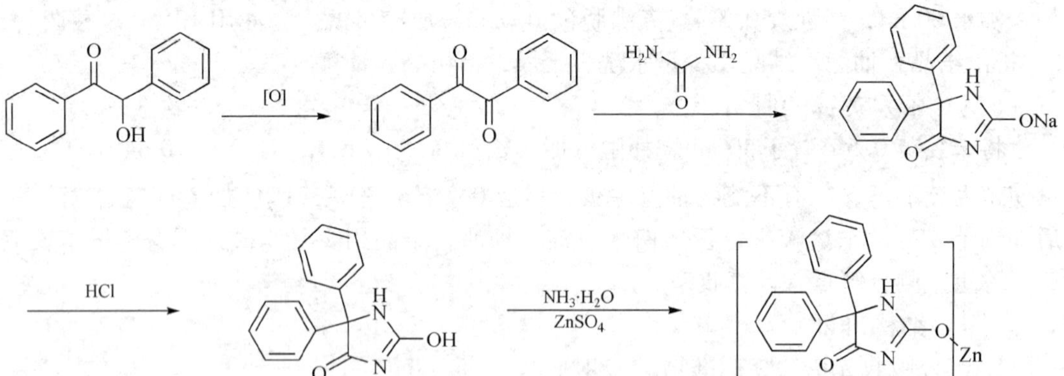

Experimental method

1. preparation of dibenzoyl

In a 250ml round-bottle flask equipped with a condenser，14 g of $FeCl_3 \cdot 6H_2O$，15 ml of ice acetic acid，6 ml of water and a grain of zeolite are added，heat on an asbestos meshwork till boil. After cooling for a while，add 2. 5 g of benzoin and a grain of zeolite，and then heat to boil for 50 min. After cooling，add another 50ml of water and a grain of zeolite, and then pour the mixture into a 250 ml beaker after heat to boil again, whisk and cooling, and separate out yellowness solid, then sieve it. Ish the crystal with a little water, dry and get the crude product. Measure its melting point, m. p. : 88-90℃, and calculate the yield.

2. Preparation of Phenytoin

In a 100ml round-bottle flask fitted with a condenser, 2 g of dibenzoyl, 15 ml of ice acetic acid, 6 ml of water, and a grain of zeolite are added, heating and refluxing for 30 minutes, then add boiling 60 ml of water, 0. 3 g of activated carbon, decolorization for 10 minutes, cooled and filtrated . The filtrate is adjusted to pH 6 with 10 % hydrochloric acid. The crystal is separated and filtrated. Ish the crystal with a little water, dry, get the crude product, and calculate the yield.

3. Preparation of Phenytoin Zinc

Put Phenytoin 0. 5 g in a 50 ml beaker, then add ammonia (including 15ml NH_3 H_2O and 10ml H_2O), let the Phenytoin dissolved, sieve out the undissolved substances. Taking another 0. 3g $ZnSO_4$ dissolve in 3 ml water and then add to the ammonia Phenytoin solution, separate out the white deposition, sieve it. Ish the crystal with a little water, dry, get the Phenytoin Zinc, weigh it, measure its decomposed point and calculate the yield.

4. Identification

(1) Infrared absorption spectroscopy; TLC counterpoint with standard substance;

(2) Nuclear magnetic resonance spectroscopy

Notes

1. It is heating with fire to boiling when preparation of dibenzoyl, and control the quality by measure the melting point.

2. The decomposed point of Phenytoin Zinc is rather high, so you should pay more attention to observe.

Questions

1. During the preparation of dibenzoyl oxidation using benzoin, what else agents can be used as oxidants? What about acidic potassium permanganate?

2. Try to state the rearrangment mechanism of benzilic acid.

3. Why do not utilize the Phenytoin which is prepared in the 2nd step to react with $ZnSO_4$, but rather synthesize the Phenytoin Zinc by changing the Phenytoin Sodium into Phenytoin, and then reacted with ammonia and zinc sulfate?

实验六 苯妥英钠（Phenytoin Sodium）的合成

【目的要求】

1. 学习安息香缩合反应的原理和应用氰化钠及维生素 B_1 为催化剂进行反应的实验方法。

2. 了解剧毒药氰化钠的使用规则。

【实验原理】

苯妥英钠为抗癫痫药，适于治疗癫痫大发作，也可用于三叉神经痛，及某些类型的心律不齐。

化学名：5,5-二苯基乙内酰脲钠。

化学结构式：

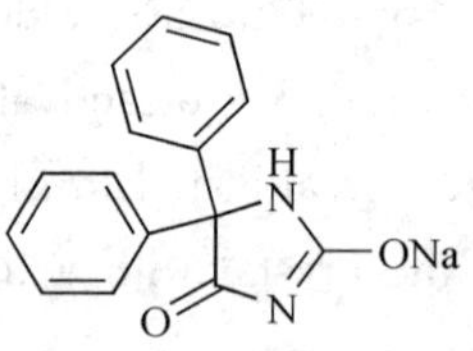

苯妥英钠为白色粉末，无臭、味苦。微有吸湿性，易溶于水，能溶于乙醇，几乎不溶于乙醚和三氯甲烷。

合成路线如下：

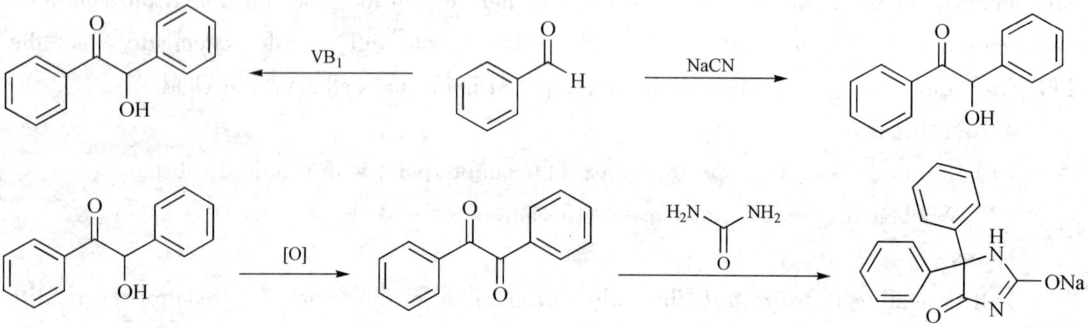

【实验方法】

(一) 安息香的制备

A 法：在装有搅拌、温度计、球型冷凝器的 100 ml 三颈瓶中，依次投入苯甲醛 12 ml，乙醇 20 ml。用20% NaOH 调至 pH 8，小心加入氰化钠 0.3 g，开动搅拌，在水浴上加热回流 1.5 h。反应完毕，充分冷却，析出结晶，抽滤，用少量水洗，干燥，得安息香粗品。

B 法：于锥形瓶内加入维生素 $B_1$2.7 g、水 10 ml、95% 乙醇 20 ml。不时摇动，待维生素 B_1溶解，加入 2mol/L NaOH 7.5 ml，充分摇动，加入新蒸馏的苯甲醛 7.5 ml，放置一周。抽滤得淡黄色结晶，用冷水洗，得安息香粗品。

(二) 联苯甲酰的制备

在装有搅拌、温度计、球型冷凝器的 100 ml 三颈瓶中，投入安息香 6 g，稀硝酸（HNO_3: H_2O = 1 : 0.6）15 ml。开动搅拌，用油浴加热，逐渐升温至 110℃ ~120℃，反应 2 h（反应中产生的氧化氮气体，可从冷凝器顶端装一导管，将其通入水池中排出）。反应毕，在搅拌下，将反应液倾入 40 ml 热水中，搅拌至结晶全部析出。抽滤，结晶用少量水洗，干燥，得粗品。

（三）苯妥英的制备

在装有搅拌、温度计、球型冷凝器的100 ml三颈瓶中，投入联苯甲酰4 g，尿素1.4 g，20% NaOH 12 ml，50% 乙醇20 ml，开动搅拌，直火加热，回流反应30 min。反应完毕，反应液倾入到120 ml沸水中，加入活性炭，煮沸10 min，放冷，抽滤。滤液用10% 盐酸调至pH 6，放置析出结晶，抽滤，结晶用少量水洗，得苯妥英粗品。

（四）成盐与精制

将苯妥英粗品置100 ml烧杯中，按粗品与水为1∶4之比例加入水，水浴加热至40℃，加入20% NaOH至全溶，加活性碳少许，在搅拌下加热5 min，趁热抽滤，滤液加氯化钠至饱和。放冷，析出结晶，抽滤，少量冰水洗涤，干燥得苯妥英钠，称重，计算收率。

（五）结构确证

1. 红外吸收光谱法、标准物TLC对照法。

2. 核磁共振光谱法。

［注释］

1. 氰化钠为剧毒药品，微量即可致死，故使用时应严格遵守下列规则：①使用时必须戴好口罩、手套，若手上有伤口，应预先用胶布贴好。②称量和投料时，避免撒落它处，一旦撒出，可在其上倾倒过氧化氢溶液，稍过片刻，再用湿抹布抹去即可。粘有氰化钠的容器、称量纸等要按上法处理，不允许不加处理乱丢乱放。③投入氰化钠前，一定要用20% NaOH调至pH 8，pH低，可产生剧毒的氰化氢气体（氰化氢为无色气体，空气中最高允许量为10 ppm）。

2. 硝酸为强氧化剂，使用时应避免与皮肤，衣服等接触，氧化过程中，硝酸被还原产生氧化氮气体，该气体具有一定刺激性，故须控制反应温度，以防止反应激烈，大量氧化氮气体逸出。

3. 制备钠盐时，水量稍多，可使收率受到明显影响，要严格按比例加水。

【思考题】

1. 试述NaCN及维生素B_1在安息香缩合反应中的作用（催化机理）。

2. 制备联苯甲酰时，反应温度为什么要逐渐升高？氧化剂为什么不用硝酸，而用稀硝酸？

3. 本品精制的原理是什么？

Experiment 6　Synthesis of Phenytoin Sodium

Purpose

1. To study the principle of benzoin condensation reaction and the experimental method which is catalyzed with vitamin B_1.

2. To learn the use regulations of sodium cyanide, a rank poison.

Mechanism

Phenytoin Sodium can be used as an antiepileptic for the treatment of grand mal epilepsy and trifacial neuralgia or some arrhythmia. Phenytoin Sodium is also named as 5,5-diphenylhydantoin Sodium, whose structure is:

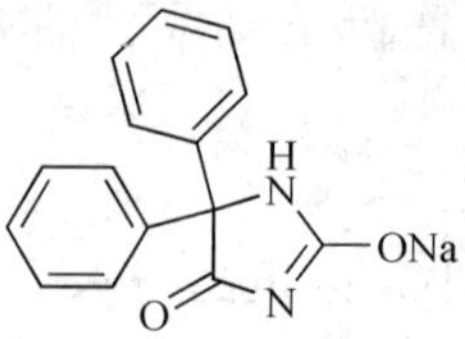

Phenytoin Sodium is a white powder, odorless, bitter in taste, blue with hygroscopicity, mp. 222-227℃ (dec.), which is soluble in water and ethanol, but hardly soluble in chloroform and ether.

The synthesis route is below:

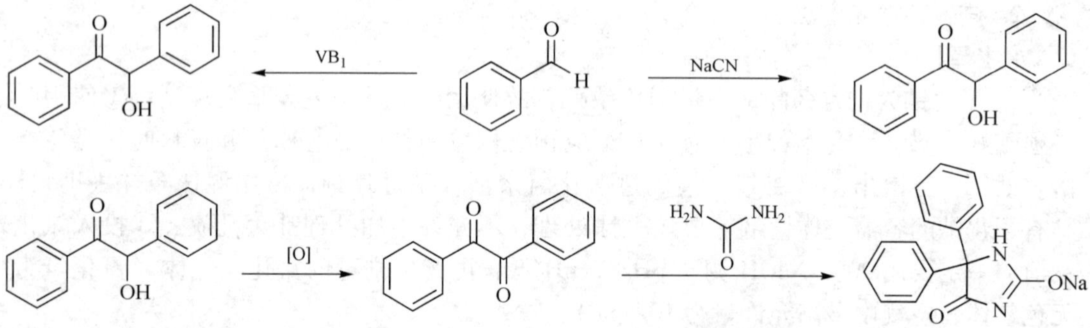

Experimental method

1. Preparation of benzoin

Method A: In a 100 ml three-necked bottle equipped with a stir bar, a thermometer and a condenser add benzaldehyde 12 ml and ethanol 20 ml in sequence. Adjust the solution to pH 8 with 20% NaOH, and add sodium cyanide 0. 3 g with caution. Stir the solution. And heat for reflux for 1. 5 h in the water bath. After the reaction complete, cooling it sufficiently and the crystal is separated out. Sieve the crystal and ish it with a small amount of water, then dry and get the crude benzoin.

Method B: Add VB_1 2. 7g, water 10 ml and 95% ethanol 20 ml in a conical flask. Shake the conical flask occasionally till VB_1 dissolve, add 2N NaOH 7. 5 ml, shake it sufficiently, and then added fresh distilled benzaldehyde, place for a week. Sieve it, and get a wheat crystal. Ish with water and get the crude benzoin.

2. Preparation of dibenzoyl

In a 100ml round – bottle flask equipped with a stir bar, a thermometer and a condenser, benzoin 6 g and dilute nitric acid (HNO_3: H_2O = 1 : 0. 6) 15 ml are added. Stir the solution, heating to 110-120℃ for 2 h in an oil bath (the gaseous NO produced in the reaction will be ejected to a water pool through a canula equipped onto the condenser. Pour the reaction mixture into 40 ml of hot water with stirring till the crystal is separated completely after the reaction being accomplished. Sieve the crystal, and ish it with a small amount of water, dry, and get the crude product.

3. Preparation of Phenytoin

In a 100ml round – bottle flask equipped with a stir bar, a thermometer and a condenser, dibenzoyl 4 g, urea 1. 4 g, 20% NaOH 12 ml and 50% ethanol 20 ml are added. Stirred the solution. And heated to reflux for 2 h with fire. Poured the reaction liquid into 120 ml of hot water after the reaction accomplished, then added active carbon and boiled for 10 min. Cooled and sieved it. Adjusted the filtrate to pH 6 with 10% hydrochloric acid, placed it to separate out the crystal, sieve it, and ish it with a small amount of water, and get the crude Phenytoin.

4. Salification and refinement

Put the crude Phenytoin into a 100ml beaker, added 4 times of water, heating to 40℃ in a water bath, and added 20% NaOH till the solid dissolved completely. Added a little active carbon, heating for 5 min with stirring, sieved it while heating, and then added sodium chloride into the filtrate to saturation. Cooled, then Separated the crystal, sieved it, ished it with a small amount of icy – water. Dried and got the Phenytoin Sodium. Weighed it and calculated the yield.

5. Identification

① Infrared absorption spectroscopy; TLC counterpoint with standard substance;

② Nuclear magnetic resonance spectroscopy.

Notes

1. Sodium cyanide is a toxicant which can lead people to death with just a little amount, so we should strictly abide the following rules when use it: ① put on the respirator and glove when use it. If there is a wound, you should paste the wound with rubberized fabric before hand. ② Avoid scattering the Sodium cyanide when weigh and use it. You should pour some hydrogen peroxide solution if you scatter it, and after a while bolt out it with a wet rag. The containers and weighing paper should be treated with as above, and do not allow to throw it out without treatment. ③ One must adjust the solution to pH 8 with 20% NaOH, for the virulent gas, hydrocyanic acid, will come into being (hydrocyanic acid is a colorless gaseous , which be allowed to no more than 10 ppm in the air) .

2. Nitric acid is a stronger oxidant which should not be contacted with skin, clothes and other things. Nitric acid will be reduced and produce NO (a gas) which has a certainty thrill in the course of oxidation, so you should control the reaction temperature in order to prevent the reaction too severely and transgress too much NO gas.

3. A little excessively water will obviously affect the yield in preparation of the sodium salt, so you should add the water strictly.

Questions

1. Try to state the function of NaCN and VB_1 in the condensation reaction of benzoin (mechanism of catalysis).

2. Why should the reaction temperature be hoisted gradually during the preparation of benzoin? Why not use nitric acid but dilute nitric acid for oxidizer?

3. What is the principle of the Phenytoin Sodium's refinement?

实验七　苯佐卡因（Benzocaine）的合成

【目的要求】

1. 通过苯佐卡因的合成，了解药物合成的基本过程。
2. 掌握氧化、酯化和还原反应的原理及基本操作。

【实验原理】

苯佐卡因为局部麻醉药，外用为撒布剂，用于手术后创伤止痛，溃疡痛，一般性痒等。

化学名；4-氨基苯甲酸乙酯

化学结构式：

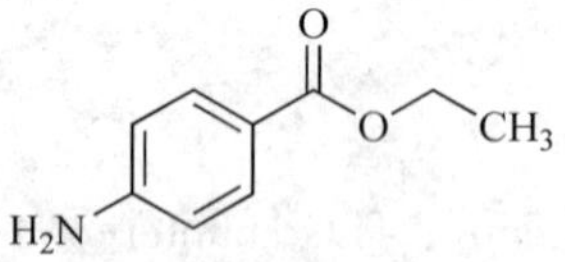

苯佐卡因为白色结晶性粉末，味微苦而麻；mp. 88℃～90℃；易溶于乙醇，极微溶于水。

合成路线如下：

路线一：

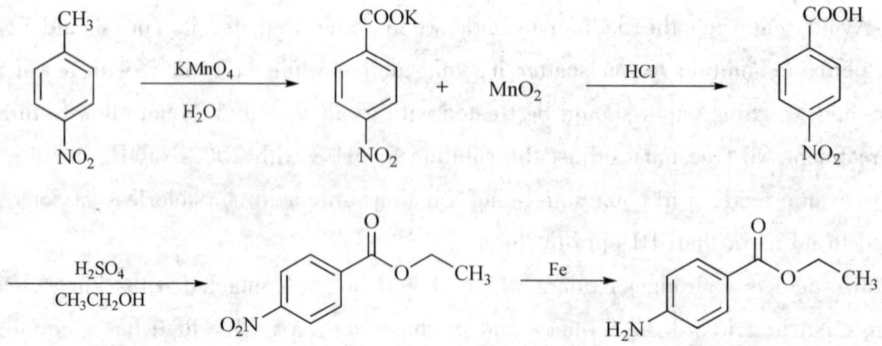

路线二：

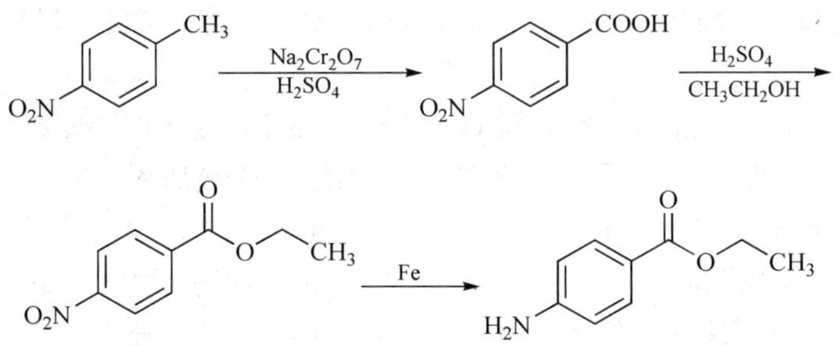

【实验方法】

（一）对硝基苯甲酸的制备（氧化）

A 法：在装有搅拌子、温度计、回流冷凝管的 250 ml 三颈瓶中，加入对硝基甲苯 7 g、高锰酸钾 10 g 及水 100 ml，开动搅拌，装上回流冷凝器，在沸水浴上加热至 80℃ 反应 1 h，加入高锰酸钾 5 g，反应 1 h 后再加入高锰酸钾 5 g，反应 0. 5h 后升温至水浴沸腾，继续反应直到高锰酸钾的颜色完全消失。如果不消失，可以加入适量亚硫酸氢钠破坏剩余的高锰酸钾。冷却至室温，抽滤，20 ml 水洗涤滤饼一次，滤液在搅拌下加浓盐酸 10 ml 酸化，待析出的沉淀冷却至室温后抽滤，水洗滤饼，抽干得产品，熔点：236℃ ~238℃，产品以乙醇为溶剂重结晶得精品（熔点可达 239℃）。

B 法：在装有搅拌棒和球型冷凝器的 250 ml 三颈瓶中，加入重铬酸钠（含两个结晶水）23. 6 g，水 50 ml，开动搅拌，待重铬酸钠溶解后，加入对硝基甲苯 8 g，用滴液漏斗滴加 32 ml 浓硫酸。滴加完毕，直火加热，保持反应液微沸 60 ~ 90 min（反应中，球型冷凝器中可能有白色针状的对硝基甲苯析出，可适当关小冷凝水，使其熔融）。冷却后，将反应液倾入 80 ml 冷水中，抽滤。残渣用 45 ml 水分三次洗涤。将滤渣转移到烧杯中，加入 5% 硫酸 35 ml，在沸水浴上加热 10 min，并不时搅拌，冷却后抽滤，滤渣溶于温热的 5% 氢氧化钠溶液 70 ml 中，在 50℃左右抽滤，滤液加入活性炭 0. 5 g 脱色（5 ~ 10 min），趁热抽滤。冷却，在充分搅拌下，将滤液慢慢倒入 15% 硫酸 50 ml 中，抽滤，洗涤，干燥得本品，计算收率。

（二）对硝基苯甲酸乙酯的制备（酯化）

在干燥的 100 ml 圆底瓶中加入对硝基苯甲酸 6 g，无水乙醇 24 ml，逐渐加入浓硫酸 2 ml，振摇使混合均匀，装上附有氯化钙干燥管的球型冷凝器，油浴加热回流 80 min（油浴温度控制在 100℃ ~120℃）；稍冷，将反应液倾入到 100 ml 水中，抽滤；滤渣移至乳钵中，研细，加入 5% 碳酸钠溶液 10 ml（由 0. 5 g 碳酸钠和 10 ml 水配成），研磨 5 min，测 pH 值（检查反应物是否呈碱性），抽滤，用少量水洗涤，干燥，计算收率。

（三）对氨基苯甲酸乙酯的制备（还原）

A 法：在装有搅拌棒及球型冷凝器的 250 ml 三颈瓶中，加入 35 ml 水，2. 5 ml 冰醋酸和已经处理过的铁粉 8. 6 g，开动搅拌，加热至 95℃ ~98℃ 反应 5 min，稍冷，加入对硝基苯甲酸乙酯 6 g 和 95% 乙醇 35 ml，在激烈搅拌下，回流反应 90 min。稍冷，在搅拌下，分次加入温热的碳酸钠饱和溶液（由碳酸钠 3 g 和水 30 ml 配成），搅拌片刻，立即抽滤（布氏漏斗需预热），滤液冷却后析出结晶，抽滤，产品用稀乙醇洗涤，干燥得粗品。

B 法：在装有搅拌棒及球形冷凝器的 100 ml 三颈瓶中，加入水 25 ml，氯化铵 0.7 g，铁粉 4.3 g，直火加热至微沸，活化 5 min。稍冷，慢慢加入对硝基苯甲酸乙酯 5 g，充分激烈搅拌，回流反应 90 min。待反应液冷至 40℃左右，加入少量碳酸钠饱和溶液调至 pH 7 ~ 8，加入 30 ml 三氯甲烷，搅拌 3 ~ 5 min，抽滤；用 10 ml 三氯甲烷洗三颈瓶及滤渣，抽滤，合并滤液，倾入 100 ml 分液漏斗中，静置分层，弃去水层，三氯甲烷层用 5% 盐酸 90 ml 分 3 次萃取，合并萃取液（三氯甲烷回收），用 40% 氢氧化钠调至 pH 8，析出结晶，抽滤，得苯佐卡因粗品，计算收率。

（四）精制

将粗品置于装有球形冷凝器的 100 ml 圆底瓶中，加入 10 ~ 15 倍（ml/g）50% 乙醇，在水浴上加热溶解。稍冷，加活性炭脱色（活性炭用量视粗品颜色而定），加热回流 20 min，趁热抽滤（布氏漏斗、抽滤瓶应预热）。将滤液趁热转移至烧杯中，自然冷却，待结晶完全析出后，抽滤，用少量 50% 乙醇洗涤两次，压干，干燥，测熔点，计算收率。

（五）结构确证

1. 红外吸收光谱法、标准物 TLC 对照法。
2. 核磁共振光谱法。

[注释]

1. 氧化反应一步在用 5% 氢氧化钠处理滤渣时，温度应保持在 50℃左右，若温度过低，对硝基苯甲酸钠会析出而被滤去。

2. 酯化反应须在无水条件下进行，如有水进入反应系统中，收率将降低。无水操作的要点是：原料干燥无水；所用仪器、量具干燥无水；反应期间避免水进入反应瓶。

3. 对硝基苯甲酸乙酯及少量未反应的对硝基苯甲酸均溶于乙醇，但均不溶于水。反应完毕，将反应液倾入水中，乙醇的浓度降低，对硝基苯甲酸乙酯及对硝基苯甲酸便会析出。这种分离产物的方法称为稀释法。

4. 还原反应中，因铁粉比重大，沉于瓶底，必须将其搅拌起来，才能使反应顺利进行，故充分激烈搅拌是铁酸还原反应的重要因素。A 法中所用的铁粉需预处理，方法为：称取铁粉 10 g 置于烧杯中，加入 2% 盐酸 25 ml，在石棉网上加热至微沸，抽滤，水洗至 pH 5 ~ 6，烘干，备用。

【思考题】

1. 氧化反应完毕，将对硝基苯甲酸从混合物中分离出来的原理是什么？
2. 酯化反应为什么需要无水操作？
3. 铁酸还原反应的机理是什么？
4. 试比较此反应中两种氧化剂的优劣。

Experiment 7 Synthesis of Benzocaine

Purpose

1. Through the synthesis of benzocaine to comprehend the elementary process of drug synthesis.

2. To master the theory and elementary operation of oxidation, esterification and reduction.

Mechanism

Benzocaine is a local anesthetic and also usually a consperative for external use. It's used for alleviating pains after operation, ulcer pain, generality itch and so on.

The chemical name of benzocaine is ethyl-4-aminobenzoate, and the structure is:

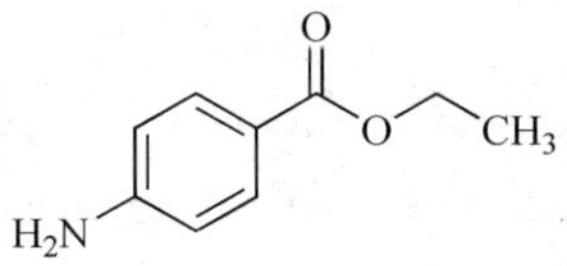

Benzocaine is a white crystalline power and has a mildly bitter flavor and felt paralyzed, mp 88-90℃, dissolve in ethanol but very slightly soluble in water.

The synthetic route 1:

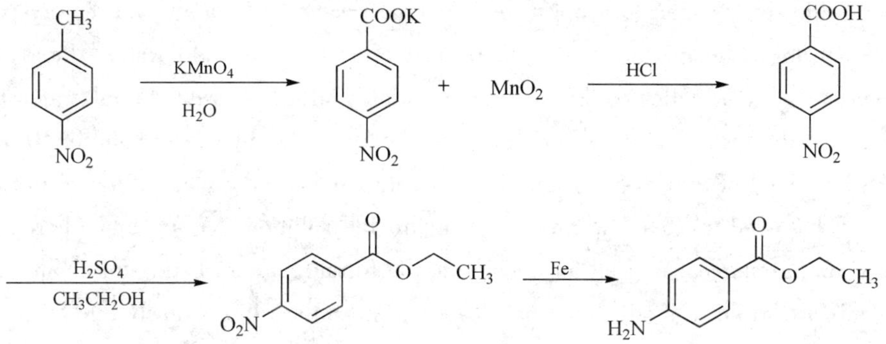

The synthetic route 2:

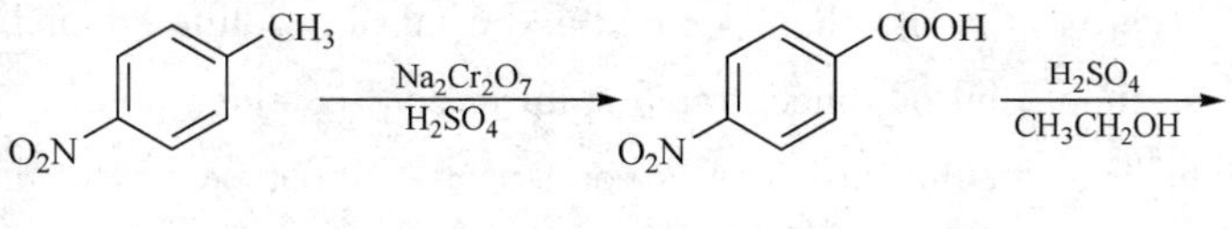

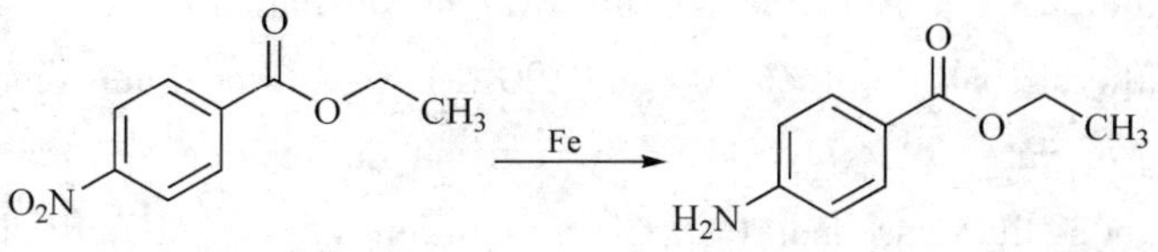

Experimental method

1. Preparation of *p*-nitrobenzoic acid (Oxidation)

Method A: Place 7 g of *p*-nitrotoluene, 10 g of potassium hypermanganate and 100 ml of water (H_2O) in a 250 ml three-neck flask equipped with a mechanical stirrer and a condenser-Allihn type. Start the mechanical stirrer (control the remote carefully) and heat to 80℃ over boiling water-bath for 1h, add 5 g of potassium hypermanganate, add another 5 g of potassium hypermanganate after 1h, the water bath is warmed to boil 30min later, the reaction continues until the color of potassium permanganate disappeared. If the colour does not disappear you can add a amount of sodium bisulfite to destroy the remaining potassium permanganate. Cool to room temperature, filter, ish the filter cake with water, 10 ml of concentrated hydrochloric acid is added in the filtrate with stirring. After crystallization precipitates completely, filtering, pressure dryness, measure weight and calculate yield. Ethanol is used as recrystallization solvent.

Method B: Place 23.6 g of sodium dichromate ($Na_2Cr_2O_7 . 2H_2O$) and 50 ml of water (H_2O) in a 250 ml three-neck flask equipped with a mechanical stirrer and a condenser-Allihn type. Start the mechanical stirrer (control the remote carefully) and then add 8g of *p*-nitrotoluene to the solution of sodium dichromate and then 32 ml of concentrated sulfuric acid is added dropwise to the mixture. After that, heat the reaction mixture briefly to gentle boiling for 60-90 min. (When reaction is processing, some *p*-nitrotoluene maybe crystallized on the condenser-Allihn type, then turn down the condensed water moderately and the crystal can be melted). Cool down the mixture and then pour it into 80 ml of cold water, then the crude *p*-nitro benzoic acid is collected by suction filtration and ish it with 45 ml water for three times. Transmit the residue to a beaker, and then heat over boiling water-bath for 10 min while agitating with 35 ml of dilute (5%) sulfuric acid solution. Cool down and filter again. The product is then dissolved in 70 ml warm sodium hydroxide solution (5%), and filtered again at about 50℃. 0.5g charcoal is used for decoloring the filtrate, after heating for about 5-10 min, filter the mixture while it's still hot. Cool down and pour the filtrate slowly into 50 ml of 15% H_2SO_4 (aq.) with continuous stir. Filter and ish the product. Dry and calculate the yield.

2. Preparation of ethyl-*p*-nitrobenzoate (Esterification)

Method A: Place 6g of *p*-nitro benzoic acid and 6 ml of absolute ethanol in a 100 ml dry, round-bottomed flask then 2 ml of concentrated sulfuric acid is added slowly. Shake the mixture until well distributed. Then fit the flask with a condenser-Allihn type with a drying tube containing calcium chloride ($CaCl_2$). Heat the mixture over an oil-bath to reflux for 80 min (control the temperature of the oil-bath between 100 and 120℃). Cool down and then pour the reaction mixture into 100 ml of water (H_2O) and filter. Transmit the residue to a mortar and comminute it, then add 10 ml of sodium carbonate (Na_2CO_3) solution (5%) (prepared by 0.5g of Na_2CO_3 and 10 ml of H_2O) and grind for 5 min. Check the pH (to detect whether the reactant is alkaline). Filter and ish with water, in a 250 ml three-neck flask fitted with a mechanical stirrer and a condenser-Allihn type. Stir the mixture and heat for 5 min(95-98℃). Cool down and then add 6 g of ethyl-p-nitro benzoate and 35 ml of ethanol (95%) into the mixture. Heated to reflux for 90 min with violent stir. Cool the solution for a few minutes and then add warm saturated solution of Na_2CO_3 fractionally (prepared by 3 g of Na_2CO_3 and 30 ml of H_2O). Stir for a moment and quickly filter the mixture(The butcher's filter needs to be warmed before). Let the filtrate cool down until the crystal separated completely, then filter it again and ish the crystal with diluted ethanol (aq). Dry the crude product.

Method B: Place 25 ml of water, 0.7 g of ammonium chloride (NH_4Cl) and 4.3 g of *pulvis aci* in a 100 ml three-neck flask fitted with a mechanical stirrer and a condenser-Allihn type. Heat the mixture to gently boiling for 5 min (Activation). Cool down and then add into 5 g of ethyl-*p*-nitro benzoate slowly. Reflux for 90 min with violent stir and cool down the reaction mixture to 40℃, then add a small amount of saturated solution of Na_2CO_3 to adjust the pH to 7 – 8. Then pour 30 ml of chloroform ($CHCl_3$) into the mixture and stir for 3 5 min. Filter and use another 10 ml of $CHCl_3$ to ish the flask and the residue. Filter again and combine the filtrate. Put it into a 100 ml Separatory funnel, let it stand and desert the water-layer. Then the $CHCl_3$-layer is also extracted by 90 ml of 5% hydrochloric acid (HCl) solution for three times. Combine the HCl(aq.)-layers (recycle the $CHCl_3$), then using 40% NaOH(aq) to adjust the pH to 8. Crystal would appear and then be filtered to collect the crude product of Benzocaine.

3. Purification

Place the crude product in a 100ml round-bottomed flask fitted with a condenser-Allihn type. Add excess (10 – 15ml/g) ethanol (50%, aq.) and then heat over a water-bath to let it dissolve. Cool down and put into some activated carbon. (The dosage of activated carbon is determined by the color of the crude product). Reflux for 20 min and then filter the mixture (The butcher's funnel and filter flask all need to be warmed before). Quickly transmit the warm filtrate to a beaker and allow the filtrate to cool slightly until crystals all have been separated. Filter and ish with a small amount of ethanol(30%, aq.)for twice. Allow the product to dry, weigh it and determine the melting point, and then calculate the yield.

4. Identification

① Infrared absorption spectroscopy.

② Nuclear magnetic resonance spectroscopy.

Notes

1. In the oxidation reaction, 5% NaOH (aq.) is used to treat the residue, and the temperature of mixture must be controlled about 50℃; if below, the sodium benzoate maybe crystallized and filtered away.

2. Esterification reaction must be operated under anhydrous condition. If water gets into the reaction system, the yield would be decreased. The key point of anhydrous operation is: the ingredient (raw material) must be anhydrous and so does the instrument and measuring appa-

ratus; during the reaction, water must be avoided ingressing into the flask.

3. Ethyl-4-nitrobenzoate and some *p*-nitrobenzoic acid (not reacted) can be dissolved in ethanol but neither in water. So when the reaction is completed, pour the reaction mixture into water(H_2O), then the concentration of ethanol would be decreased and *p*-nitrobenzoic acid would be crystallized. This method of separation is named as Dilution Method.

4. In the reduction reaction, the density of *pulvis aci* is large and would be placed at the bottom. So must stir them up and then the reaction can perform rightly. In a word, violent stir is the key factor of the reduction reaction. In the method A, the *pulvis aci* has to be pretreated: place 10 g of *pulvis aci* in a beaker, then add 25 ml of HCl (2%, aq.), heat to gentle boiling, filter and ish it with water to pH 5 - 6, then dry it by oven and store it for use.

Questions

1. When the oxidation reaction is completed, what is the theory of separating p - nitrobenzoic acid from the mixture?

2. Why does the esterfaction reaction need anhydrous operation?

3. What is the mechanism of the reduction reaction?

4. Try to compare the advantages and disadvantages between the two oxidants.

实验八　磺胺嘧啶锌（Sulfadiazine-Zn）与磺胺嘧啶银（Sulfadiazine-Ag）的合成

【目的要求】

了解拼合原理在药物结构修饰中的应用。

【实验原理】

磺胺嘧啶银为应用烧伤创面的磺胺药，对铜绿假单胞菌有强的抑制作用，其特点是保持了磺胺嘧啶与硝酸银二者的抗菌作用。用于治疗烧伤创面感染和控制感染外，还可使创面干燥，结痂，促进愈合。但磺胺嘧啶银成本较高，且易氧化变质，故制成磺胺嘧啶锌，以代替磺胺嘧啶银。

化学名：2-(对氨基苯磺酰胺基)嘧啶银(SD-Ag)

2-(对氨基苯磺酰胺基)嘧啶锌(SD-Zn)

化学结构式：

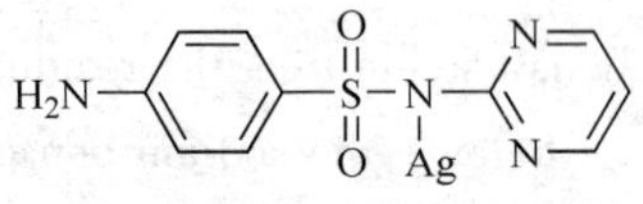

SD-Ag

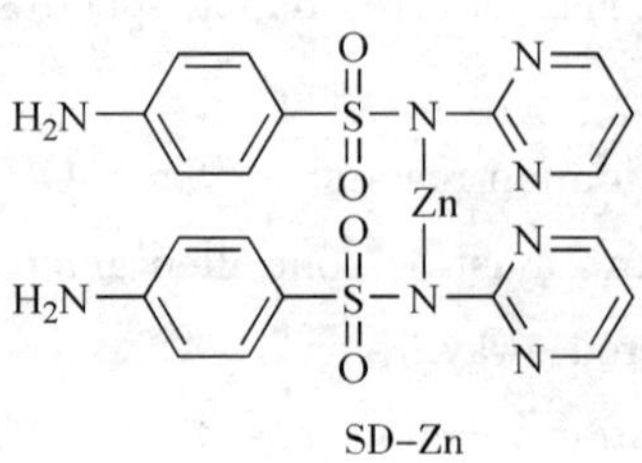

SD-Zn

磺胺嘧啶银为白色或类白色结晶性粉末，遇光或遇热易变质。在水、乙醇、三氯甲烷或乙醚中均不溶。磺胺嘧啶锌为白色或类白色粉末，在水、乙醇、三氯甲烷、或乙醚中均不溶。

合成路线如下：

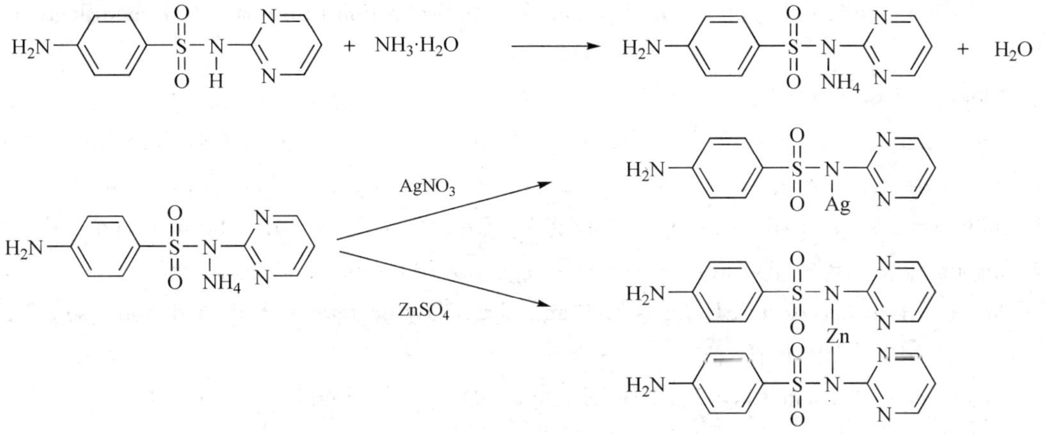

【实验方法】

（一）磺胺嘧啶银的制备

取磺胺嘧啶 5 g，置 50 ml 烧杯中，加入 10% 氨水 20 ml 溶解。再称取 $AgNO_3$ 3. 4 g 置 50 ml 烧杯中，加 10 ml 氨水溶解，搅拌下，将 $AgNO_3$ - 氨水溶液倾入磺胺嘧啶 - 氨水溶液中，片刻析出白色沉淀，抽滤，用蒸馏水洗至无 Ag^+ 反应，得本品。干燥，计算收率。

（二）磺胺嘧啶锌的制备

取磺胺嘧啶 5 g，置 100 ml 烧杯中，加入稀氨水（4 ml 浓氨水加入 25 ml 水），如有不溶的磺胺嘧啶，在补加少量浓氨水（约 1 ml 左右）使磺胺嘧啶全溶。另称取硫酸锌 3 g，溶于 25 ml 水中，在搅拌下倾入上述磺胺嘧啶氨水溶液中，搅拌片刻析出沉淀，继续搅拌 5 min，过滤，用蒸馏水洗至无硫酸根离子反应（用 0. 1 M 氯化钡溶液检查），干燥，称重，计算收率。

（三）结构确证

1. 红外吸收光谱法、标准物 TLC 对照法。
2. 核磁共振光谱法。

［注释］

合成磺胺嘧啶银时，所有仪器均需用蒸馏水洗净。

【思考题】

1. SD - Ag 及 SD - Zn 的合成为什么都要先作成铵盐？
2. 比较 SD - Ag 及 SD - Zn 的合成及临床应用方面的优缺点。

Experiment 8 Synthesis of Sulfadiazine-Zn and sulfasiazine-Ag

Purpose

To comprehend the application of principle of hybridization in the structure modification of drugs.

Mechanism

Sulfadiazine-Ag is a sulfa drug applied for burn wound, it displays powerful inhibitory action to *aeruginosus Bacillus*. Its feature is that it retains both the antibacterial activity of Slufapyrimidine (SD) and silver nitrate ($AgNO_3$). Except used for curing burn wound and controlling infection, it's also applied for making raw surface dry and scab which can promote concrescent. But the cost of SD-Ag is high and also easily degenerated by oxidation, so SD-Zn is synthesized to replace SD-Ag.

Their chemical name is: 2-sulfanilyl amino SD-Ag, 2-sulfanilyl amino SD-Zn.

The structure is:

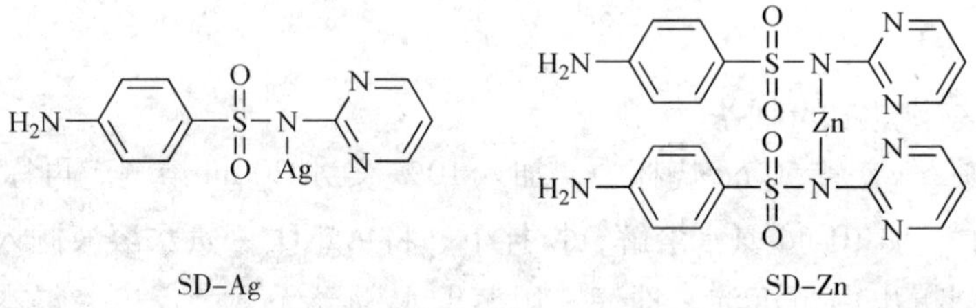

SD-Ag is a white or off-white color crystalline powder, and easily degenerated by light or heat. It's dissoluble in water, ethanol, chloroform and ethyl ether. SD-Zn is also white or off-white color crystalline powder; the character of its solubility is the same as SD-Ag.

Synthesis route:

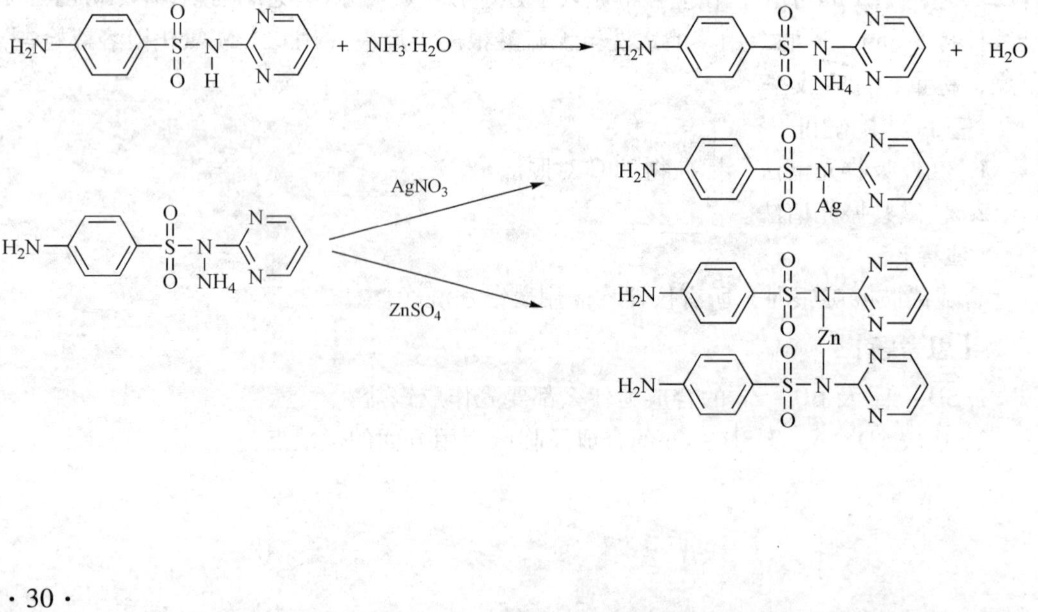

Experiment Method

1. Preparation of SD-Ag

Place 5 g of Sulfapyrimidine into a 50ml beaker, then add 20 ml of 10% aqueous ammonia ($NH_3 \cdot H_2O$) to dissolve it and set it aside. Place 3. 4 g of silver nitrate ($AgNO_3$) in another 50 ml beaker and get 10 ml of $NH_3 \cdot H_2O$ to dissolve it. With Stirring, pour $AgNO_3$ – $NH_3 \cdot H_2O$ solution into the SD-$NH_3 \cdot H_2O$ solution. A moment later, white precipitate would appear then filtered and ished with water until no Ag^+ reaction processed. Then dry the product and calculate the yield.

2. Preparation of SD-Zn

5 g of Sulfapyrimidine is placed into a 100ml beaker, then some diluted ammonia water ($NH_3 \cdot H_2O$) (prepared by 4 ml of aqueous ammonia and 25 ml of water) is added to dissolve it. If some SD still doesn't dissolve, add about 1 ml of aqueous ammonia to make the SD all dissolved. Get 3g of zinc sulfate ($ZnSO_4$) dissolved in 25 ml of water and with stirrig, pour the solution to the SD-$NH_3 \cdot H_2O$ solution, a moment later, precipitate would appear then stir for another 5 min and filtered, ished with water until no SO_4^{2-} reaction processed (tested with 0. 1 M barium chloride ($BaCl_2$)). Dry, weigh it and calculate the yield.

3. Identification

① Infrared absorption spectroscopy; TLC counterpoint with standard substance.

② Nuclear magnetic resonance spectroscopy.

Notes

When synthesizing SD-Ag, all instruments should be cleaned with distilled water.

Questions

1. Why should SD-Ag and SD-Zn be transformed to their amine salt fistly in the synthesis?

2. Compare the advantage and disadvantage between SD-Ag and SD-Zn, in the aspect of synthesis procedure and clinical application?

实验九 琥珀酸喘通（Clorprenaline Succinate）的合成

【目的要求】

了解拼合原理在药物结构修饰中的应用。

【实验原理】

止喘药喘通为β_2-受体兴奋剂，对游离组胺、乙酰胆碱等神经化学介质引起的支气管痉挛有良好的缓解作用，但能使一些患者出现心悸、手颤等症状。盐酸喘通体内代谢快，12h 即从尿排除 80% ~90%。为了克服以上副作用并使药效缓和而持久，依据文献关于琥珀酸有平喘作用的报导，将盐酸喘通制成琥珀酸喘通。

化学名：1-(邻氯苯基)-2-异丙胺基乙醇丁二酸盐

化学结构式：

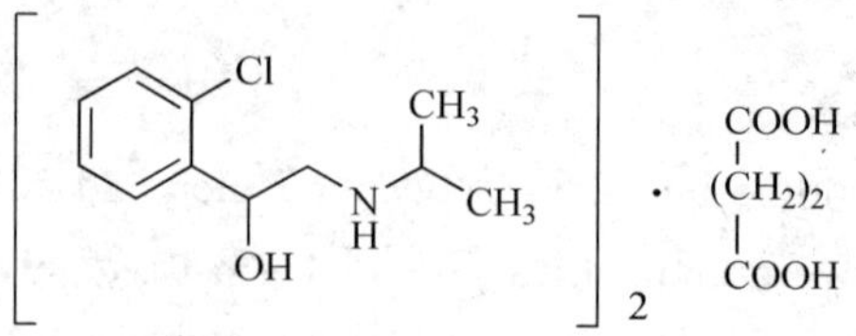

琥珀酸喘通为无色透明的菱形结晶。无臭，味微苦。极易溶于水，易溶于乙醇，难溶于乙醚、丙酮。mp. 171. 5℃ ~173℃。

合成路线如下：

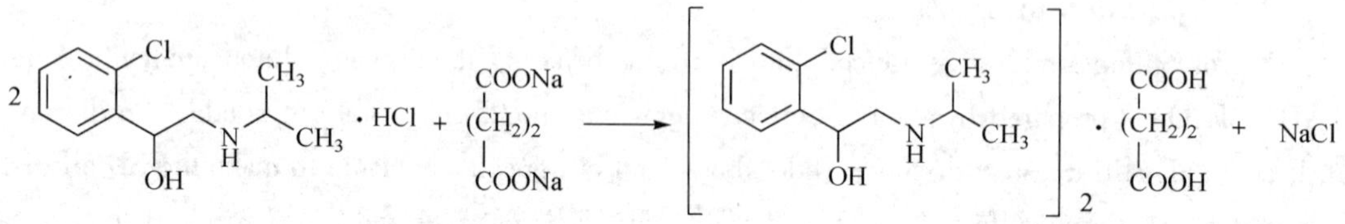

【实验方法】

（一）琥珀酸喘通的制备

称取盐酸喘通 4. 5 g，溶于 5 ~7 ml 水中，置水浴中温热，制成饱和溶液。另称取琥珀酸钠 4. 9 g 溶于 5 ml 水中，制成饱和溶液。然后，在不断搅拌下，将盐酸喘通溶液加入琥珀酸钠溶液中，慢慢析出琥珀酸喘通盐结晶，抽滤，结晶用 10 ml 水分两次迅速洗涤，干燥，测熔点，计算收率。

（二）结构确证

1. 红外吸收光谱法、标准物 TLC 对照法。
2. 核磁共振光谱法。

［**注释**］盐酸喘通、琥珀酸喘通极易溶于水，故反应中要严格控制用水量。

【思考题】

1. 为何将盐酸喘通制成琥珀酸喘通？这一设计思想对药物修饰有何启示？
2. 琥珀酸喘通结晶为什么要用水迅速洗涤？不洗是否可以？

Experiment 9 Synthesis of Cloprenaline Succinate

Purpose

To understand the application of hybridization in the structure modification.

Mechanism

The powerful bronchodilator Clorprenaline is an β_2-agonist, which can excellently release the convulsion of bronchia caused by neuro – medium, such as isolated histamine and acetylcholine. But it also causes side-effects in some patients, for example, heart-throb, hand-tremble. Clorprenaline hydrochloride can be easily metabolized in vivo, and 80%-90% is eliminated in urine after 12 hours. In order to overcome these side-effects and make it slowlier release and hold the effect long, linked to that succinic acid is also a bronchodilator, Clorprenaline succinate is synthesized.

Its chemical name is: 1-(2-Chloro-1-phenyl)-2-isopropylaminoethanol succinate.

Chemical structure is as follows:

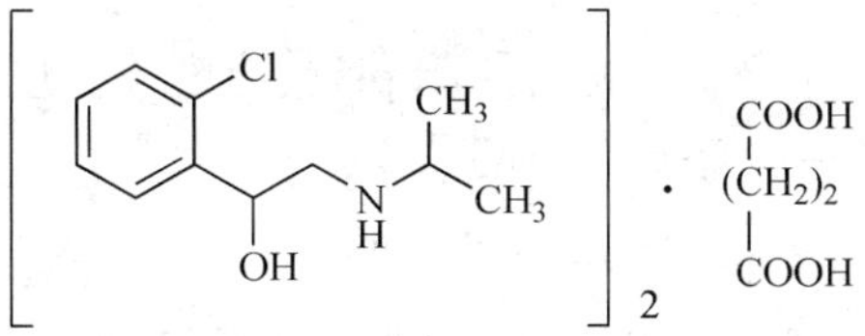

Physical chemistry property of Clorprenaline succinate: colourless diomand crystal, odorless and slightly bitter. Easily dissolve in water, easy in ethanol, insoluble in ether and acetone, mp. 171.5-173℃.

The synthetic route

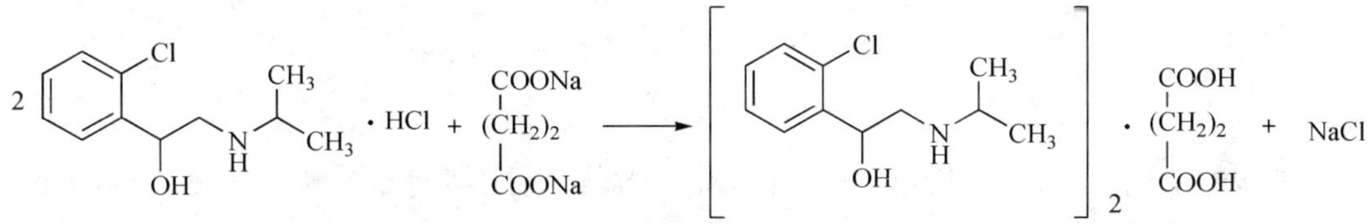

Experiment Method

1. Preparation of Clorprenaline Succinate

4.5 g of Cloprenaline Hydrochloride is dissolved in 5 to 7ml of water, then put them in a water bath to gain its saturated solution. At the same time, 4.9 g of sodium succinate is dissolved in 5 ml of water to gain its saturated solution. Then the cloprenaline solution is added to sodium succinate solution under stirring, and the crystal of Clorprenaline Succinate slowly grows up. The crystal is filtrated and quickly ished by 10 ml of water for 2 times, then dried, and measure its mp, calculate the yield.

2. Identification

① Infrared absorption spectroscopy; TLC counterpoint with standard substance.

② Nuclear magnetic resonance spectroscopy.

Note

Because that Cloprenaline Hydrochloride and Cloprenaline Succinate are easily solubale in water, the amount of water in reaction need be controlled stickly.

Questions

1. Why should Clorprenaline Hydrochloride be made into Clorprenaline Succinate? What do you learn from the design philosophy applicated in medicine structural modification?

2. Why the Cloprenaline Succinate crystal need be ished by water quickly? Could it be not ished ?

实验十 磺胺醋酰钠（Sulfacetamide Sodium）的合成

【目的要求】

1. 通过磺胺醋酰钠的合成，了解用控制 pH、温度等反应条件纯化产品的方法。
2. 加深对磺胺类药物一般理化性质的认识。

【实验原理】

磺胺醋酰钠用于治疗结膜炎、沙眼及其他眼部感染。

化学名：*N*-[(4-氨基苯基)-磺酰基]-乙酰胺钠-水合物

化学结构：

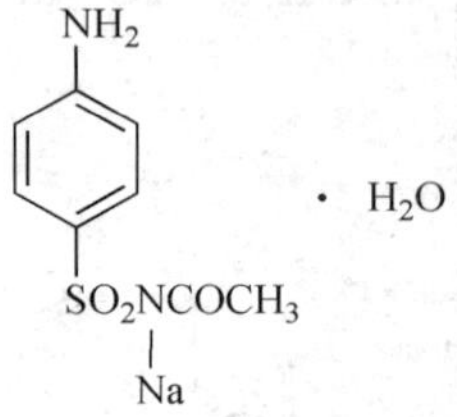

磺胺醋酰钠为白色结晶性粉末；无臭味，微苦。易溶于水，微溶于乙醇、丙酮。

合成路线如下：

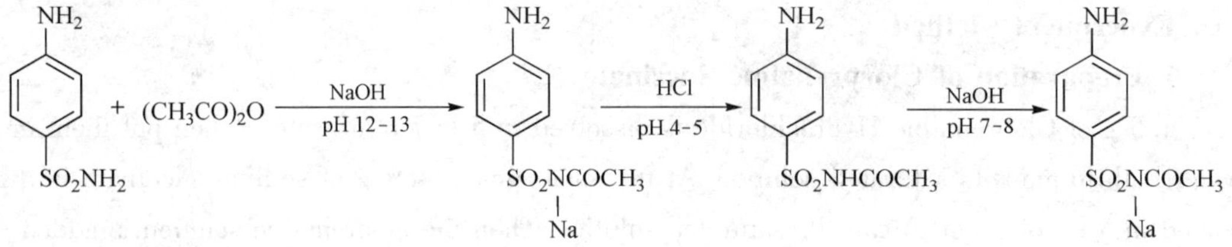

【实验方法】

（一）磺胺醋酰的制备

在装有搅拌棒及温度计的 100 ml 三颈瓶中，加入磺胺 17.2 g，22.5% 氢氧化钠 22 ml，开动搅拌，于水浴上加热至 50℃左右。待磺胺溶解后，分次加入醋酐 13.6 ml，77% 氢氧化钠 12.5 ml（首先，加入醋酐 3.6 ml，77% 氢氧化钠 2.5 ml；随后，每次间隔 5 min，将剩余的 77% 氢氧化钠和醋酐分 5 次交替加入）。加料期间反应温度维持在 50℃ ~55℃；加料完毕继续保持此温度反应 30 min。反应完毕，停止搅拌，将反应液倾入 250 ml 烧杯中，加水 20 ml 稀释，于冷水浴中用 36% 盐酸调至 pH 7，放置 30 min，并不时搅拌析出固体，抽滤除去。滤液用 36% 盐酸调至 pH 4 ~5，抽滤，得白色粉末。

用 3 倍量（3 ml/g）10% 盐酸溶解得到的白色粉末，不时搅拌，尽量使单乙酰物成盐酸盐溶解，抽滤除不溶物。滤液加少量活性炭室温脱色 10 min，抽滤。滤液用 40% 氢氧化钠调至 pH 5，析出磺胺醋酰，抽滤，压干。干燥，测熔点（mp. 179℃ ~184℃）。若产品不和格，可用热水（1∶5）精制。

（二）磺胺醋酰钠的制备

将磺胺醋酰置于 50 ml 烧杯中，于 90℃热水浴上滴加计算量的 20% 氢氧化钠至固体恰好溶解，放冷，析出结晶，抽滤（用丙酮转移），压干，干燥，计算收率。

（三）结构确证

1. 红外吸收光谱法、标准物 TLC 对照法。

2. 核磁共振光谱法。

［注释］

1. 在反应过程中交替加料很重要，以使反应液始终保持一定的 pH 值（pH 12 ~ 13）。

2. 按实验步骤严格控制每步反应的 pH 值，以利于除去杂质。

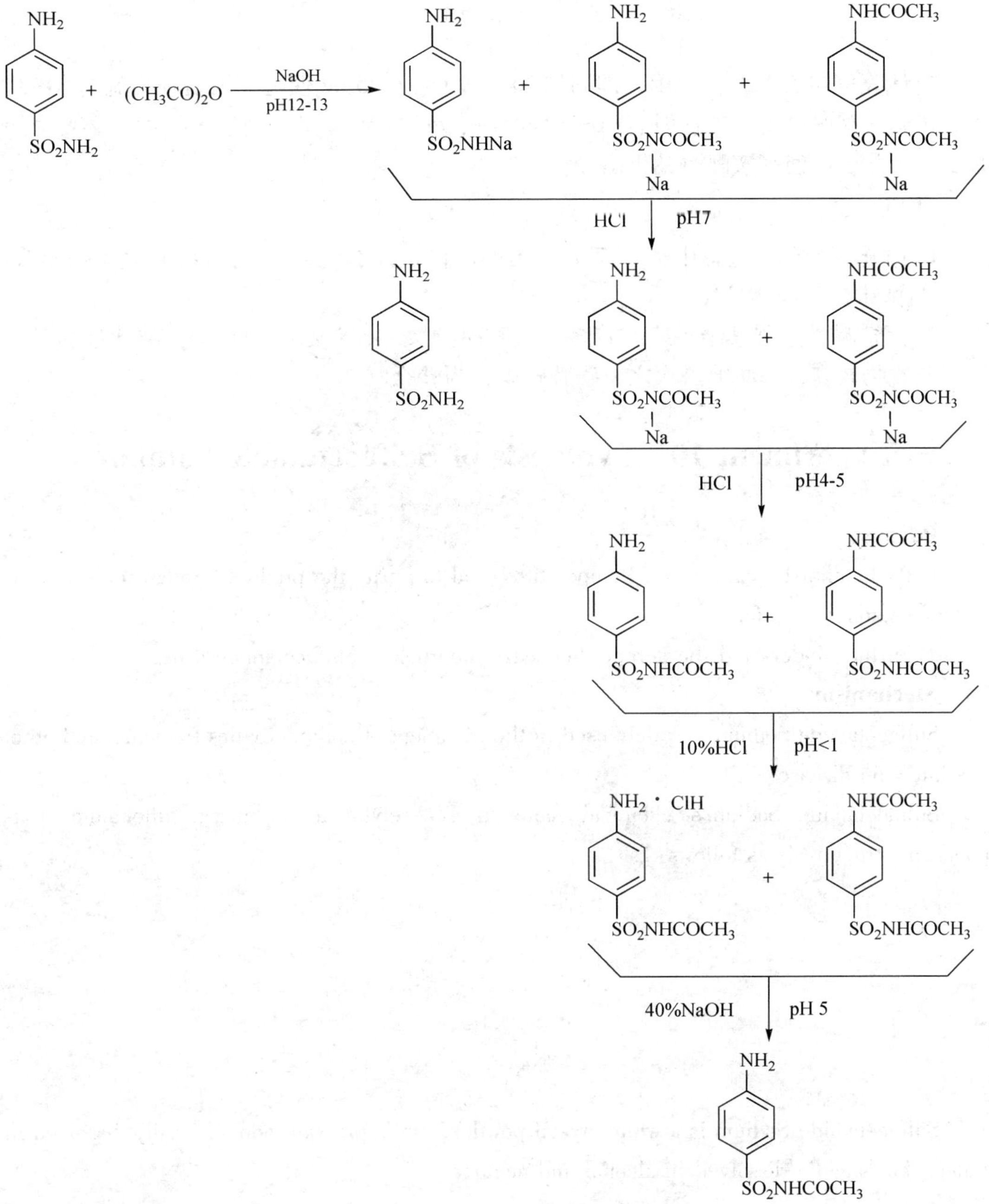

3. 将磺胺醋酰制成钠盐时，应严格控制 20% NaOH 溶液的用量，按计算量滴加。

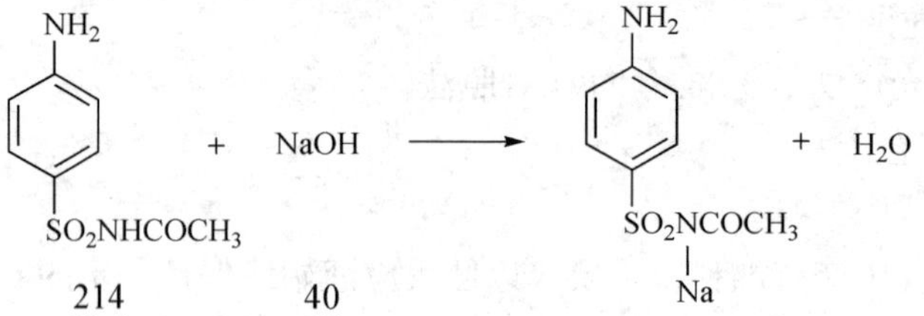

214　　40
12.5　　X

214:40=12.5:X　　X=2.3g

由计算可知需 2.3 g NaOH，即滴加 20% NaOH 11.5 ml 便可。因磺胺醋酰钠水溶性大，由磺胺醋酰制备其钠盐时若 20% NaOH 的量多于计算量，则损失很大。必要时可加少量丙酮，以使磺胺醋酰钠析出。

【思考题】

1. 酰化液处理的过程中，pH 7 时析出的固体是什么？pH 5 时析出的固体是什么？10% 盐酸中的不溶物是什么？

2. 反应碱性过强其结果磺胺较多，磺胺醋酰次之，双乙酰物较少；碱性过弱其结果双乙酰物较多，磺胺醋酰次之，磺胺较少，为什么？

Experiment 10 Synthesis of Sulfacetamide Sodium

Purpose

1. Be familiar to control pH, temperature et al to purify the product through the synthesis of Sulfacetamide Sodium.

2. Further understand the gernal chemical properties of Sulfacetamide drugs.

Mechanism

Sulfacetamide Sodium is widely used in the treatment of conjunctivities trachoma and other eye infection diseases.

Sulfacetamide Sodium's chemical name is *N*-Acetyl-4-amino-benzenesulfonamide, its chemical structure is as follows:

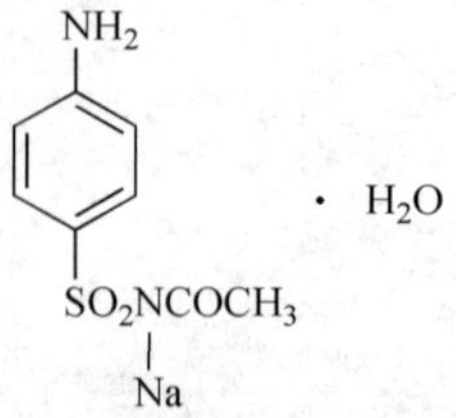

Sulfacetamide Sodium is a white crystal powder, no unpleasant odour, easily dissolved in water, but slightly dissolved in alcohol and acetone.

Following is the synthesis route:

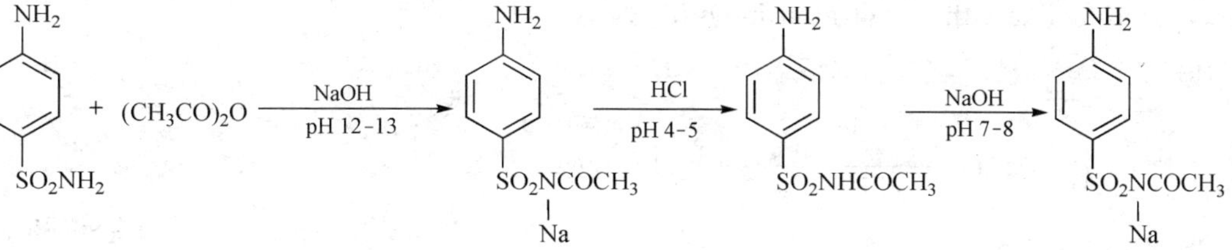

Experiment Method

1. Preparation of Sulfacetamide

In a 100ml three-neck flask charged with a stirrer and a thermometer, 17. 2 g of sulfanilamide and 22 ml of sodium hydroxide are added (22. 5%) . Then stirred in a water bath, the temperature should be controlled at about 50℃. After Sulfacetamide dissolved, 13. 6 ml of acetic anhydride and 12. 5 ml of sodium hydroxide (22. 5%) are added for several pitches (first add 3. 6 ml of acetic anhydride, then 2. 5 ml of sodium hydroxide (77%), after that every 5 min, add the remain acetic anhydride and sodium hydroxide alternately). During the enriching process, the temperature should keep 50-55℃, after all agents are added, kept this temperature for 30 minutes. When the reaction finishes , pour the reactive liquid to a 250 ml beaker, add 20 ml of water to distill it. Then use hydrochloric acid (36%) to adjust pH to 7 in an ice-water bath, keep this temperature for 30 minutes, and keep stirring. At the same time, there is crystal separated out. Remove it with filter. The filtrate is adjusted with 36% HCl to pH 4-5, then filtrate it and get white powder.

Dissolve the white powder with 3 folds of HCl (3ml/g), with continuous stirring, dissolve the monoace to chloro salt as much as possible, filtrate the insoluble agent. Add a little activated carbon to the filtrate at room temperature and decolorized for 10 minutes. The filtrate is adjusted to the pH 5 with NaOH (40%), the Sulfacetamide would crystallize from mother liquid, filtrate and dry the product, test the melt point (mp. 179-184℃), if the product is not correct, it could be refined with hot water (1 : 5) .

2. Preparation of Sulfacetamide Sodium

In a 50ml beaker charged with Sulfacetamide, dropp sodium hydroxide (20%) in 90℃ until the solid dissolved , cool it to room temperature, it will crystallize from mother liquid, filtrate it (use acetone to transfer the product), after dryness, calculate the yield.

3. Identification

① Infrared absorption spectroscopy; TLC counterpoint with standard substance.

② Nuclear magnetic resonance spectroscopy.

Notes

1. The reactants should be added alternately during the reaction in order to maintain pH 12-13.

2. The pH in each step must be controlled strictly according to the experimental procedure in order to facilitate the removal of impurities.

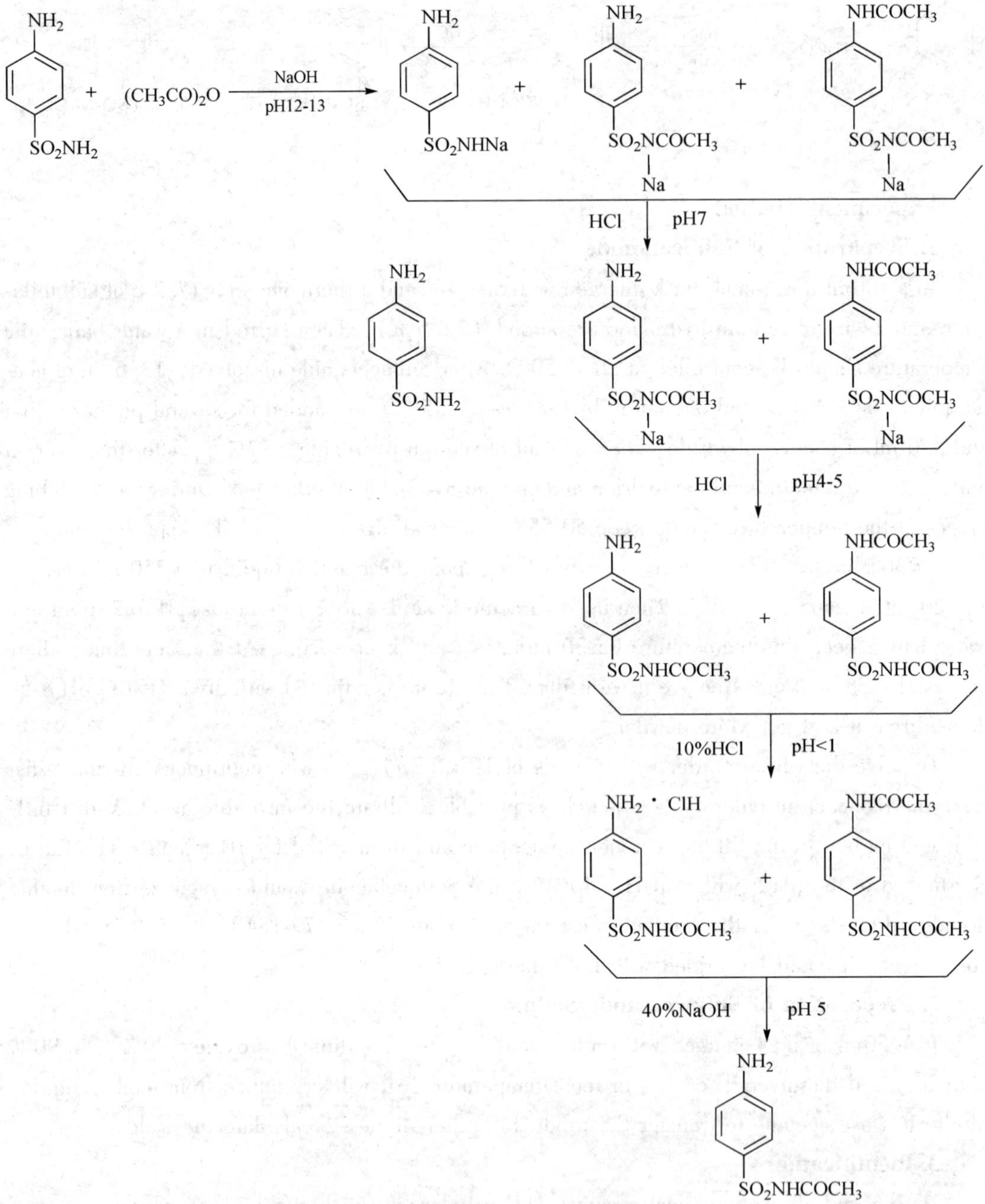

3. The amount of 20% NaOH should be controlled strictly and dropped according to the calculation when sulfacetamide is transformed to be Sulfacetamide Sodium.

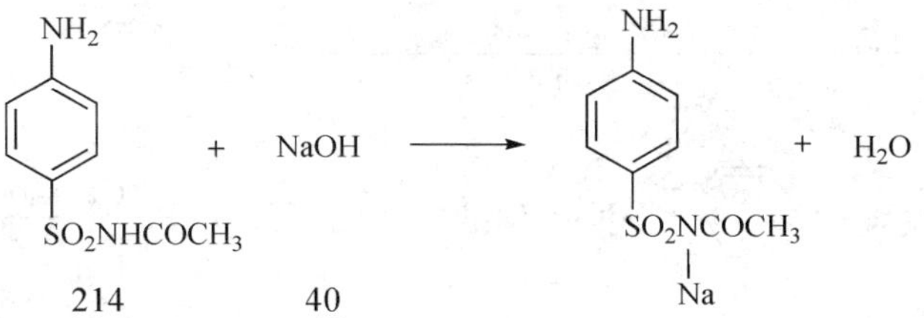

214　　40
12.5　　X

214:40=12.5:X　　X=2.3g

2.3 g of NaOH (namely 11.5 ml of 20% NaOH) is required according to the calculation above. Because sulfacetamide sodium is easy to dissolve in water, if the amount of 20% NaOH is more than that of the calculation, sulfacetamide sodium will suffer from great loss. If necessary, a small amount of acetone should be added in order to make sulfacetamide sodium separate out.

Questions

1. During treatment with acylation solution, what is the precipitated solid when pH = 7? When pH = 5? What is the insoluble agent in 10% HCl?

2. Too strong alkaline will result in more sulfonamides, followed by sulfacetamide, and diacetyl derivatives the least; too weak alkaline will result in more diacetyl derivatives, followed by sulfacetamide, and sulfonamides the least. Try to state the reason.

实验十一 盐酸普鲁卡因（Procaine Hydrochloride）的合成

【目的要求】

1. 通过局部麻醉药盐酸普鲁卡因的合成，学习酯化、还原等单元反应。
2. 掌握利用水和二甲苯共沸脱水的原理进行羧酸的酯化操作。
3. 掌握水溶性大的盐类用盐析法进行分离及精制的方法。

【实验原理】

盐酸普鲁卡因为局部麻醉药，作用强，毒性低。临床上主要用于浸润、脊椎及传导麻醉。

化学名：对氨基苯甲酸2-二乙胺基乙酯盐酸盐

化学结构式：

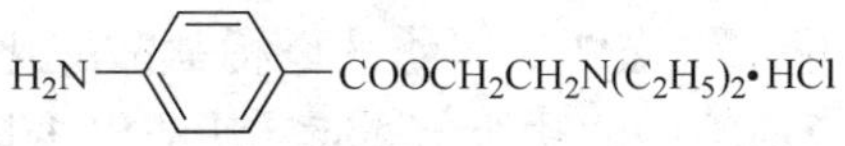

盐酸普鲁卡因为白色细微针状结晶或结晶性粉末，无臭，味微苦而麻。熔点153℃～157℃。易溶于水，溶于乙醇，微溶于三氯甲烷，几乎不溶于乙醚。

合成路线如下：

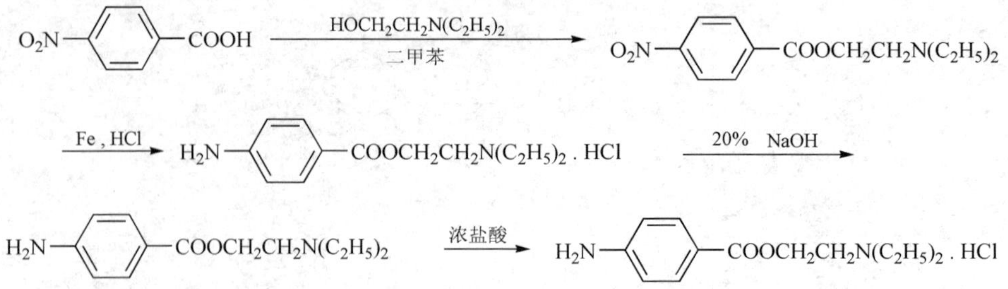

【实验方法】

(一) 对硝基苯甲酸-β-二乙胺基乙醇(俗称硝基卡因)的制备

在装有温度计、分水器及回流冷凝器的500 ml三颈瓶中，投入对硝基苯甲酸20 g、β-二乙胺基乙醇14.7 g、二甲苯150 ml及止爆剂，油浴加热至回流(注意控制温度，油浴温度约为180℃，内温约为145℃)，共沸带水6 h。撤去油浴，稍冷，将反应液倒入250 ml锥形瓶中，放置冷却，析出固体。将上清液用倾泻法转移至减压蒸馏烧瓶中，水泵减压蒸除二甲苯，残留物以3% 盐酸140 ml溶解，并与锥形瓶中的固体合并，过滤，除去未反应的对硝基苯甲酸，滤液(含硝基卡因)备用。

[注释]

(1) 羧酸和醇之间进行的酯化反应是一个可逆反应。反应达到平衡时，生成酯的量比较少(约65.2 %)，为使平衡向右移动，需向反应体系中不断加入反应原料或不断除去生成物。本反应利用二甲苯和水形成共沸混合物的原理，将生成的水不断除去，从而打破平衡，使酯化反应趋于完全。由于水的存在对反应产生不利的影响，故实验中使用的药品和仪器应事先干燥。

(2) 考虑到教学实验的需要和可能，将分水反应时间定6 h，若延长反应时间，收率尚可提高。

(3) 也可不经放冷，直接蒸去二甲苯，但蒸馏至后期，固体增多，毛细管堵塞操作不方便。回收的二甲苯可以套用。

(4) 对硝基苯甲酸应除尽，否则影响产品质量，回收的对硝基苯甲酸经处理后可以套用。

(二) 对氨基苯甲酸-β-二乙胺基乙醇酯的制备

将上步得到的滤液转移至装有搅拌器、温度计的500 ml三颈瓶中，搅拌下用20% 氢氧化钠调pH 4.0~4.2。充分搅拌下，于25℃分次加入经活化的铁粉，反应温度自动上升，注意控制温度不超过70℃(必要时可冷却)，待铁粉加毕，于40℃~45℃保温反应2 h。抽滤，滤渣以少量水洗涤两次，滤液以稀盐酸酸化至pH 5。滴加饱和硫化钠溶液调pH 7.8~8.0，沉淀反应液中的铁盐，抽滤，滤渣以少量水洗涤两次，滤液用稀盐酸酸化至pH 6。加少量活性炭，于50℃~60℃保温反应10 min，抽滤，滤渣用少量水洗涤一次，将滤液冷却至10℃以下，用20% 氢氧化钠碱化至普鲁卡因全部析出(pH 9.5~10.5)，过滤，得普鲁卡因，备用。

［注释］

（1）铁粉活化的目的是除去其表面的铁锈，方法是：取铁粉 47 g，加水 100 ml，浓盐酸 0.7 ml，加热至微沸，用水倾泻法洗至近中性，置水中保存待用。

（2）该反应为放热反应，铁粉应分次加入，以免反应过于激烈，加入铁粉后温度自然上升。铁粉加毕，待其温度降至 45℃进行保温反应。在反应过程中铁粉参加反应后，生成绿色沉淀 $Fe(OH)_2$，接着变成棕色 $Fe(OH)_3$，然后转变成棕黑色的 Fe_3O_4。因此，在反应过程中应经历绿色、棕色、棕黑色的颜色变化。若不转变为棕黑色，可能反应尚未完全。可补加适量铁粉，继续反应一段时间。

（3）除铁时，因溶液中有过量的硫化钠存在，加酸后可使其形成胶体硫，加活性炭后过滤，便可使其除去。

（三）盐酸普鲁卡因的制备

1. 成盐 将普鲁卡因置于烧杯中，慢慢滴加浓盐酸至 pH 5.5，加热至 60℃，加精制食盐至饱和，升温至 60℃，加入适量保险粉，再加热至 65℃～70℃，趁热过滤，滤液冷却结晶，待冷至 10℃以下，过滤，即得盐酸普鲁卡因粗品。

2. 精制 将粗品置烧杯中，滴加蒸馏水至维持在 70℃时恰好溶解。加入适量的保险粉，于 70℃保温反应 10 min，趁热过滤，滤液自然冷却，当有结晶析出时，外用冰浴冷却，使结晶析出完全。过滤，滤饼用少量冷乙醇洗涤 2 次，干燥，得盐酸普鲁卡因，mp. 153℃～157℃，以对硝基苯甲酸计算总收率。

［注释］

（1）盐酸普鲁卡因水溶性很大，所用仪器必须干燥，用水量需严格控制，否则影响收率。

（2）严格掌握 pH 5.5，以免芳胺基成盐。

（3）保险粉为强还原剂，可防止芳胺基氧化，同时可除去有色杂质，以保证产品色泽洁白，若用量过多，则成品含硫量不合格。

（四）结构确证

1. 红外吸收光谱法、标准物 TLC 对照法。
2. 核磁共振光谱法。

【思考题】

1. 在盐酸普鲁卡因的制备中，为何用对硝基苯甲酸为原料先酯化，然后再进行还原，能否反之，先还原后酯化，即用对硝基苯甲酸为原料进行酯化？为什么？
2. 酯化反应中，为何加入二甲苯做溶剂？
3. 酯化反应结束后，放冷除去的固体是什么？为什么要除去？
4. 在铁粉还原过程中，为什么会发生颜色变化？说出其反应机制。
5. 还原反应结束，为什么要加入硫化钠？
6. 在盐酸普鲁卡因成盐和精制时，为什么要加入保险粉？解释其原理。

Experiment 11 Synthesis of Procaine Hydrochloride

Purpose

1. To learn the esterification, reduction and several other elemental reactions through the synthesis of local anesthetics procaine hydrochloride.

2. To grasp the esterification operation of carboxyl acid by virtue of getting rid of water through the co – boiling of water and xylene.

3. To grasp the seperation and refinement of salts with high water – solubility through a salt out.

Mechanism

Procaine hydrochloride is a local anesthetic, which has a strong effect but low toxicity. It is mostly used to soak the acantha and transmit the anaesthesia.

The chemical name of procaine hydrochloride is *p*-aminobenzoic acid 2-(diethylamino) ethyl ester hydrochloride, of which the structure is:

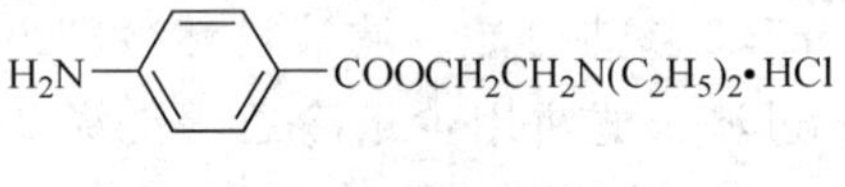

Procaine hydrochloride is a white little spiculate crystal or crystal powder, which is odorless, faintly bitter and has a benumbing taste. mp. 153-157℃. It could dissolve into water easily, and is soluble in ethanol, less soluble in chloroform, but hardly dissolve in diethyl ether.

The synthetic route is as follows:

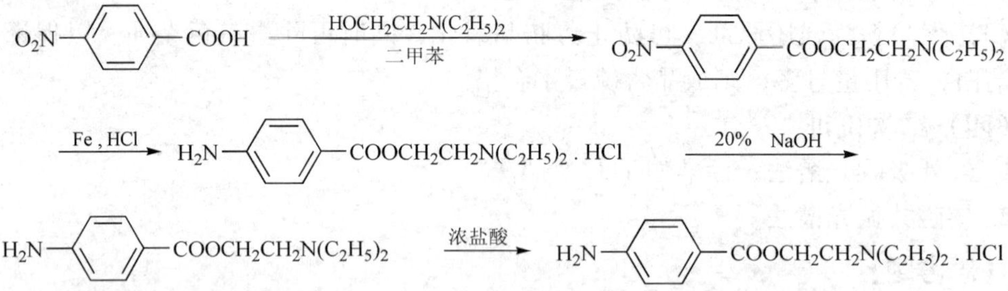

Experiment method

1. Preparation of *p*-nitrobenzoic acid-β-(diethylamino) ethyl ester

Add 20 g of *p*-nitrobenzoic acid, 14.7 g of β-(diethylamino) ethanol, 150ml of xylene and anti-blast agent to a 500 ml three-necked flask installed with thermometer, trap for water and condenser, heat to reflux in an oil bath (pay attention to control the temperature, the outside temperature is 180℃, but 145℃ inside), getting rid of water by co-boiling for 6h. Remove the oil bath and cool, pour the reactant solvent into a 250 ml conical flask, lay and cool to separate the solid. Pour the top solvent into a distilled flask, evaporate the xylene under reduced-pressure by water pump. The residue is dissolved with 140 ml of 3% hydrochloride acid, which is combined with the solid in the conical flask, filtered to remove the unreacted *p*-nitrobenzoic acid, the filtrate (containing *p*-nitrobenzoic acid-β-(diethylamino) ethyl ester is on standby.

Notes:

(1) The esterification between carboxyl acid and alcohol is a reverse reaction. When reaching the equilibrium, the amount of produced ester is little (ca. 65.2%), in order to transform the equilibrium to the right, it is necessary to add reagents or remove the product continuously. In this reaction, by virtue of the co-boiling of water and xylene, the produced water is removed continuously, thereby transformed the equilibrium, which mostly completed the reaction. Because of the adverse effect of water, the reagents and apparatus used in the experiment are all needed to be dried beforehand.

(2) Considering the need and probability in teaching experiment, the time to seperate water is choosen to be 6 h, if longer, the yield will increase.

(3) It is not allowed to evaporate the xylene directly without cooling, but at the end of distillation, the solid increased to block the capillary, which resulted in unconvenience. The reclaimed xylene could be recycled .

(4) It is necessary to remove up the *p*-nitrobenzoic acid, which affects the quality of the product. The reclaimed *p*-nitrobenzoic acid could be recycled.

2. Preparation of *p*-aminobenzoic acid 2-(diethylamino) ethyl ester

Add the filtrate prepared in last step to a 500ml three-necked flask with a stirrer and a thermometer, adjust the pH 4.0-4.2 with sodium hydroxyl under stirring. Under well stirring, the activated ferrous powder is added in batches, the temperature of reactant would raise automatically. Pay attention to control the temperature below 70℃ (it is necessary to cool sometimes). After adding, react at 40-45℃ for 2 h. Filtrate, ish the residue twice with a little amount of water, acidify the filtrate to pH 5 with diluted hydrochloride acid. Drop the saturated sodium sulfide solvent and adjust the pH 7.8-8.0, in order to make the ferrous salts in the solvent deposited. Filtrate and ish the residue twice with a little amount of water, acidify the filtrate to pH 6 with diluted hydrochloride acid. A little active carbon is added, then react at 50-60℃ for 10mins. Fitrate, ish the residue once with little amount of water, cool the filtrate below 10℃ , which is basified with sodium hydroxyl until all the procaine separated out (pH 9.5-10.5) . Fitrate and gain the procaine on standby.

Notes

(1) The activation of the ferrous powder is to remove the rust on the surface. Methods: to dissolve 47 g of ferrous powder with 100 ml of water, 0.7 ml of concentrated hydrochloride acid, heat to a bit boiling state, then ish with pouring water to neutral. The product is deposited in the water on standby.

(2) Because of the heat-produced reaction, the ferrous powder should be added in batches to prevent a blast reaction. The temperature raised spontaneously after the addition of fer-

rous powder, however, the temperature-controlled reaction should start when the temperature fell down to 45℃. During the reaction the ferrous powder turned to a green solid $Fe(OH)_2$, then the brown $Fe(OH)_3$ and the black Fe_3O_4 finally. Thus a color transformation from green to brown and black in the end occurred in the reaction. If the black color did not occur, the reaction might not have completed. Additional ferrous powder should be added to continue the reaction for longer time.

(3) During the removing of ferrous powder, the excess sodium sulfide would form a sulphur after the addition of acid, the activated carbon should be added to remove the colloid of sulphur through filtration.

3. Preparation of Procaine Hydrochloride

(1) Salts formation Add the procaine to a beaker, then drop the concentrated acid to pH 5. 5 slowly, heat to 60℃, saturate with refined sodium chloride. Heat to 60℃, then sodium dithionite is added. Heat to 65-70℃ again, fitrate while the solvent is hot. Cool the filtrate to crystallize. When the temperature fell down to 10℃, filtrate and gain the crude of Procaine Hydrochloride.

(2) Refinement Add the crude to a beaker, drop the distilled water just to dissolve the solid at 70℃. Add sodium dithionite and react at 70℃ for 10mins. Filtrate while the solvent is hot. Cool the filtrate naturally. On separating out the crystal, cool it with an ice-bath to complete the crystallization. Filtrate, ish the pad twice with little cold ethanol. Dry and gain the procaine hydrochloride, mp. 153-157℃, calculate the total yield according to the *p*-nitrobenzoic acid.

Notes

(1) Because of the well solubility of procaine hydrochloride in water, all the apparatus must be dried. The amount of water used in the experiment should also be controlled, which will affect the yield.

(2) Control the pH 5. 5 to prevent the salts formation of the aromatic amino group strictly.

(3) The sodium dithionite is a strong reductant, which could prevent the oxidation of aromatic amino group and remove the colored by-product to white the product at the same time. However a excess amount would result in a disqualification.

4. Identification

① Infrared absorption spectroscopy; TLC counterpoint with standard substance.

② Nuclear magnetic resonance spectroscopy.

Questions

1. Why esterify the *p*-nitrobenzoic acid first before the reduction of ethyl *p*-nitrobenzoic in the preparation of procaine hydrochloride. Could the sequence be reverse?

2. Why is xylene added as solvent in the esterification.

3. What is the solid cooled to remove after the esterification? Why to remove it?

4. Why did a color transformation occur during the reduction with ferrous powder? Try to

explain the mechanism of the reaction.

5. Why is the sodium sulfide added after the reduction?

6. Why is the sodium dithionite added during the salts formation and refinement of procaine hydrochlorid? Try to explain the principle.

实验十二　盐酸普鲁卡因（Procaine Hydrochloride）稳定性实验

【目的要求】

1. 了解 pH 值对盐酸普鲁卡因溶液稳定性的影响。
2. 了解薄层层析法检查药物中杂质的方法。

【实验原理】

盐酸普鲁卡因为局部麻醉药，作用强，毒性低。临床上主要用于浸润、脊椎及传导麻醉。盐酸普鲁卡因化学名为对氨基苯甲酸 2-二乙胺基乙酯盐酸盐，化学结构式为：

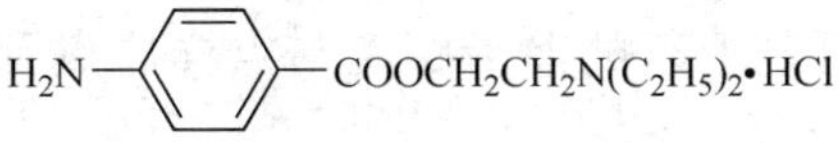

盐酸普鲁卡因为白色细微针状结晶或结晶性粉末，无臭，味微苦而麻。易溶于水，溶于乙醇，微溶于三氯甲烷，几乎不溶于乙醚。mp. 153℃～157℃。

盐酸普鲁卡因溶液不稳定，易被水解，在一定温度下，水解速度随氢氧离子浓度的增加而加快。

反应如下：

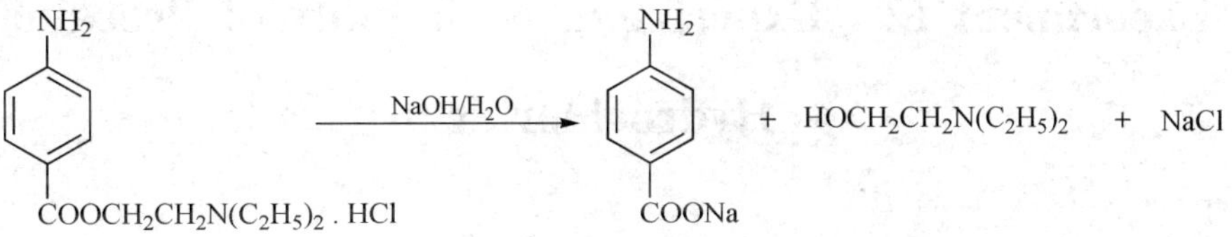

【实验方法】

（一）薄层板的制备

取层析用硅胶 GF_{254} 粉 2.5 g，加 0.5% CMC 溶液 7.5 ml，于研钵中研磨成糊状，涂铺在平滑洁净玻璃板（5 cm×20 cm）上，阴干，备用。

（二）试液的制备

1. 标准液的制备

（1）0.2% 对氨基苯甲酸溶液，作为点样液 A。

（2）0.4% 盐酸普鲁卡因溶液，作为点样液 B。

2. 供试液的制备

（1）取0.4% 盐酸普鲁卡因溶液5 ml，用0.1mol/L盐酸调至pH 2 ~ 3，沸水浴中加热25 min，倾入10 ml烧杯中，作为点样液C。

（2）取0.4% 盐酸普鲁卡因溶液5 ml，用0.1mol/L氢氧化钠调至pH 9 ~ 10，沸水浴中加热25 min，倾入10 ml烧杯中，作为点样液D。

（三）点样

在制好的薄层板上，距下端边缘2.5 cm处，分别用毛细管取点样液A、B、C、D进行点样，两点间相距1 cm，于靠边一侧相距约1 cm。

（四）展开

用丙酮与1% 盐酸（9∶1）混合液作为展开剂，置于密闭的层析槽中，待饱和30 min后，将已点样的薄层板放入，用倾斜上行法展开，展开剂上升与点样的位置相距一定距离处（一般为10 ~ 15 cm）取出薄层板，风干。

（五）显色

用对二甲氨基苯甲醛试液（对二甲氨基苯甲醛1 g，溶于30% 盐酸25 ml及甲醇75 ml混合液中）喷雾显色，或在紫外灯下看展开的斑点，用铅笔画好。

（六）计算

根据点样液原点到展开剂上行的前沿距离与点样原点到上行色点中心距离相比求出比移值（R_f 值）。

【思考题】

1. 盐酸普鲁卡因溶液的稳定性受哪些因素的影响？
2. 为什么用对二甲氨基苯甲醛试液显色？
3. 薄层色谱法在药物分析中有何用途？

Experiment 12 Experiment of Stability of Procaine Hydrochloride

Purpose

1. To learn the effects of pH on stability of Procaine Hydrochloride.
2. To learn the ways that TLC tests the impurity of drug.

Mechanism

Procaine Hydrochloride is a kind of drug of local anesthesia, strong effect and low toxicity, used in the anaesthesia of soakage, acantha and transmitting.

Its chemical name: 4-aminobenzoic acid 2-(diethyl amino)ethyl ester and the structure is as follows:

Procaine Hydrochloride, white crystals of needle or powder, slightly bitter taste, Sol. in water, alcohol, slightly sol. in chloroform, almost insol. in ether. mp. 153-157℃, instable and hydrolyzed easily. Reaction is as follows:

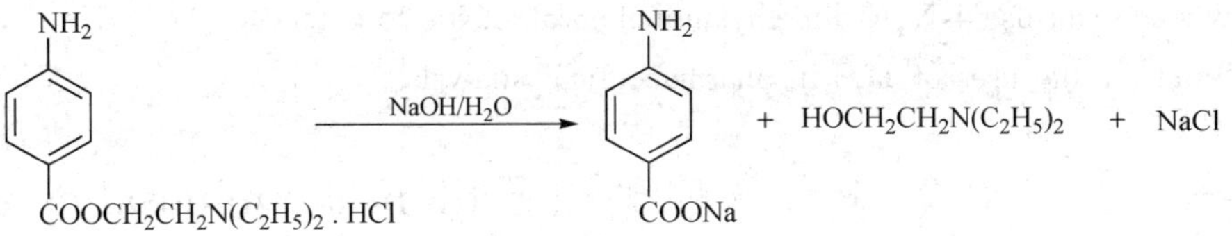

Experiment methods

1. Preparation of TLC

2.5 g of GF_{254} powder is added to 7.5 ml of 0.5% CMC, which is grinded in a mortar to a slurry and then is spread on the clean glass backing plates (5 cm × 20 cm), air-dry and wait to be used.

2. Preparation of test solution

(1) preparation of standard solution

① 0.2% 4-aminobenzoic acid as Sample A.

② 0.4% Procaine Hydrochloride as Sample B.

(2) Preparation of supplied test solution

① 5ml of 0.4% Procaine Hydrochloride is adjusted to pH 2-3 by 0.1N hydrogen chloride and then is heated in boiling water for 25 min, the solution is poured into a 10 ml of beaker, as Sample C.

② 5ml of 0.4% Procaine Hydrochloride is adjusted to pH 9-10 by 0.1N sodium hydroxide and then is heated in boiling water for 25 min, the solution is poured into a 10 ml of beaker, as Sample D.

3. Sample application

Samples A, B, C, D to be separated are applied near to the bottom of the plate (2.5cm from bottom) using the thinner capillaries. Every tow samples are away from 1cm and the first sample is away from the edge about 1cm.

4. Development

The mobile phases of acetone and 1% hydrogen chloride (9 : 1) are placed in a sealed tank and saturated for 30 mins and then the preparative plate is put into the tank until the solvent is away from the samples 10-15 cm, development is achieved, take out the plate and air-dry.

5. Detection

Spray detection: 4-*N*,*N*-dimethylbenzaldehyde is required as a spray reagent, or use UV to see spots and the spots are indicated by pencil.

6. Calculation

R_f value: according to the front distance and sample point as well as the central distance.

Questions

1. What are the factors to affect thestability of Procaine Hydrochloride?
2. Why do you use 4-N, N-dimethylaminobenzaldehyde to detect?
3. What are the uses of TLC in pharmaceutical analysis?

实验十三　对氨基水杨酸钠（Sodium *p*-Aminosalicylate）稳定性实验

【目的要求】

通过本实验，加强对实验中防止药物氧化重要性的认识。

【实验原理】

对氨基水杨酸钠（PAS-Na）用于治疗各种结核病，尤适用于肠结核、骨结核及渗出性肺结核的治疗。

化学结构式为：

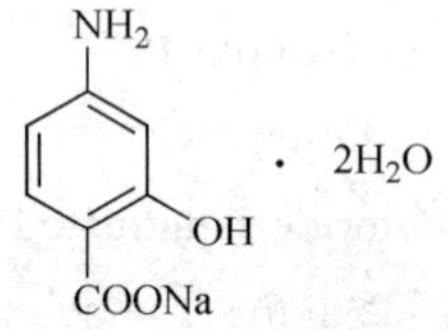

对氨基水杨酸钠为白色或银灰色结晶性粉末，mp. 142℃～145℃，难溶于水及三氯甲烷，溶于乙醇及乙醚，几乎不溶于苯。

对氨基水杨酸钠盐水溶液很不稳定，易被氧化，遇光热颜色渐变深。在铜离子存在下，加速氧化。如有抗氧剂或金属络合剂存在，可有效地防止氧化。用光电比色计测定透光率（T）可看出其变化程度。

反应如下：

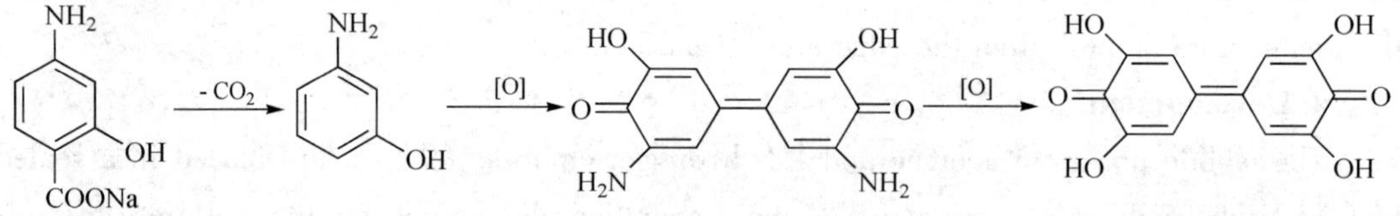

【实验方法】

取5支试管，编号，各加入0.025 % PAS-Na溶液10 ml。除1号试管外，各试管分别加入双氧水（10～50 ml）12滴。在3号试管中加入 $Na_2S_2O_5$ 试液（10 g～30 ml）20滴。在4、5号试管中分别加入 Cu^{2+} 试液（2 mg～10 ml）6滴。在5号试管加入EDTA试液（10 mg～10 ml）20滴。各试管用蒸馏水稀释至刻度一致。

将所有试管同时置入80℃～90℃水浴中，记录置入时间，维持此温度，间隔30 min取样，放置至室温，用722型分光光度计在440 nm处测定各样品的透光率。

【思考题】

1. 药物被氧化着色与哪些因素有关，如何采取措施防止药物氧化?
2. PAS-Na 氧化后生成何物？写出反应式。

Experiment 13 Stability Experiment of Sodium *p*-Aminosalicylate

Purpose

To enhance the realization of importance that avoids the oxidation of drug from this experiment.

Mechanism

PAS-Na is used to cure tuberculosis, the same with tuberculosis of intestines, bone and lung. Its structure is below:

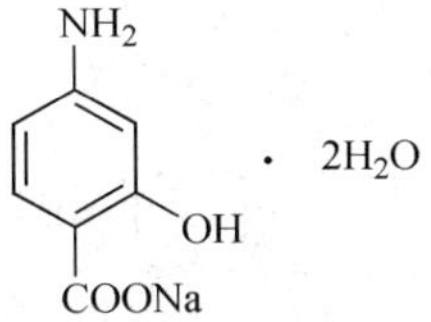

PAS-Na is a white or silver gray crystallized powder, mp. 142-145℃, dissolve difficultly in water and chloroform, dissolve in alcohol and diethyl ether, dissolve hardly in benzene

PAS-Na is instable, oxidation is happened easily, when it encounters light and hot, the color is turned deeply, when copper ion exist, the speed of oxidation is quicker than before. If the antioxidant or metallic complexing agent exists, the oxidation is avoided, according to T, the movement can be seen. The reaction is as follows:

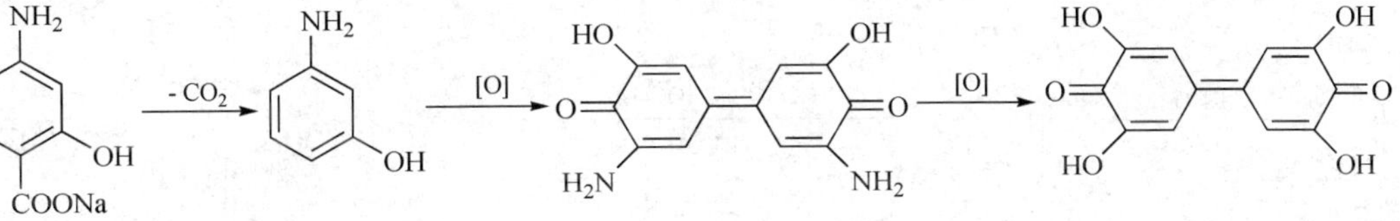

Experiment method

10ml of 0. 025% PAS-Na is added into 5 test tubes with numbers separately, except tube 1, 12 droppings of H_2O_2 (10ml-50ml) are added into the others separately, 20 droppings of $Na_2S_2O_5$ (10ml -30ml) are added into tube 3, 6 droppings of Cu^{2+} test solution (2ml -10ml) are added into tube 4, 5. 20 droppings of EDTA test solution are added into tube 5. Every tube is diluted to the same volume by distilled water.

All of the tubes are put into the water-bath (80-90℃) at the same time, note the time and maintain the temperature, after 30 mins, the samples are taken and placed to rt. and then the samples are tested the light transmittance by 722-spectrophotometer at 422nm.

Questions

1. What factors are about the oxidation and pigmentation? How to avoid them?
2. After the oxidation of PAS-Na, what reaction has happened? Write the reaction.

实验十四　二氢吡啶钙离子拮抗剂的合成

【目的要求】

1. 了解硝化反应的种类、特点及操作条件。
2. 学习硝化剂的种类和不同应用范围。
3. 学习环合反应的种类、特点及操作条件。

【实验原理】

二氢吡啶钙离子拮抗剂具有很强的扩血管作用，适用于冠脉痉挛、高血压、心肌梗死等症。本品化学名为1,4-二氢-2,6-二甲基-4-(3-硝基苯基)-吡啶-3,5-二羧酸二乙酯，化学结构式为：

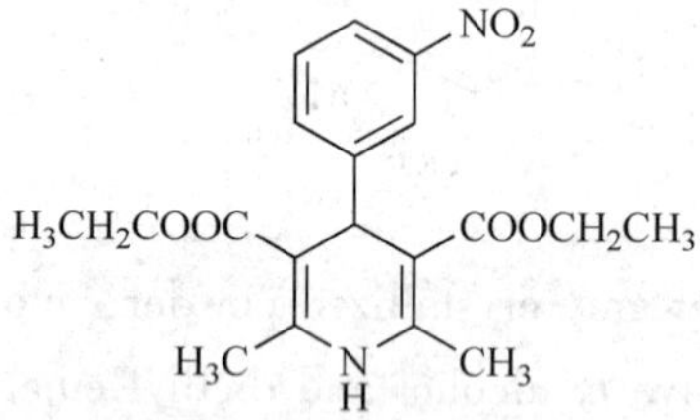

本品为黄色无臭无味的结晶粉末，mp. 162℃ ~164℃，无吸湿性，极易溶于丙酮、二氯甲烷、三氯甲烷，溶于乙酸乙酯，微溶于甲醇、乙醇，几乎不溶于水。

合成路线如下：

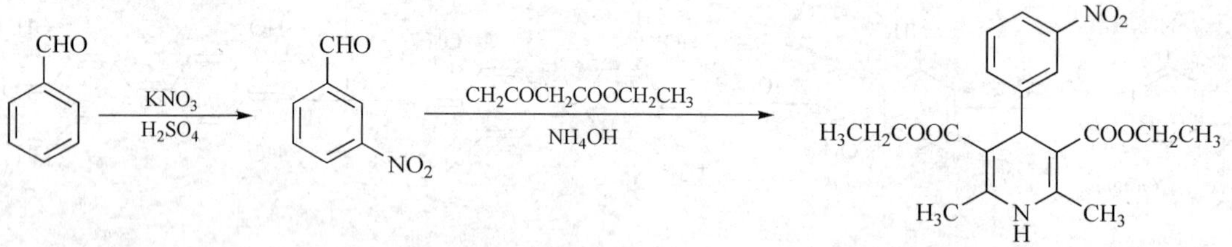

【实验方法】

(一) 硝化

在装有搅拌棒、温度计和滴液漏斗的250 ml三颈瓶中，将11 g硝酸钾溶于40 ml浓硫酸中。用冰盐浴冷至0℃以下，在强烈搅拌下，慢慢滴加苯甲醛10 g（在60 ~90 min左右滴完），滴加过程中控制反应温度在0℃ ~2℃之间。滴加完毕，控制反应温度在0℃ ~5℃之间继续反应90 min。将反应物慢慢倾入约200 ml冰水中，边倒边搅拌，析出黄色固体，抽滤。滤渣移至乳钵中，研细，加入5 % 碳酸钠溶液20 ml（由1 g碳酸钠加20 ml水配成）研磨5 min，抽滤，用冰水洗涤7 ~8 次，压干，得间硝基苯甲醛，自然干燥，测熔点（mp. 56℃ ~58℃），称重，计算收率。

（二）环合

在装有球型冷凝器 100 ml 圆底中，依次加入间硝基苯甲醛 5 g、乙酰乙酸乙酯 9 ml、甲醇氨饱和溶液 30 ml 及沸石一粒，油浴加热回流 5 h，然后改为蒸馏装置，蒸出甲醇至有结晶析出为止，抽滤，结晶用 95% 乙醇 20 ml 洗涤，压干，得黄色结晶性粉末，干燥，称重，计算收率。

（三）精制

粗品以 95% 乙醇（5ml/g）重结晶，干燥，测熔点，称重，计算收率。

（四）结构确证

1. 红外吸收光谱法、标准物 TLC 对照法。
2. 核磁共振光谱法。

［注释］

甲醇氨饱和溶液应新鲜配制。

【思考题】

1. 根据所学知识，总结硝化剂种类有哪些？及其应用范围。
2. 试解释本环合反应机理。

Experiment 14 Synthesis of Dihydropyridine Calcium Channel Blocker

Purpose

1. To comprehend the kinds, characteristics and operation conditions of nitrifying reaction.
2. To learn the kinds of nitrating agent and different ranges of applications.
3. To learn the kinds, characteristics and operated conditions of cyclization.

Mechanism

Dihydropyridine calcium channel blocker has strong enlarge blood vessel function, it is applied to treat coronary artery convulsion, hypertension and cardiac muscle death and soon.

Its chemical name is 1,4-dihydro-2,6-dimethyl-4-(3-nitro-phenyl)-3,5-pyridinedicarboxylic acid diethyl ester, and its structure is as follows:

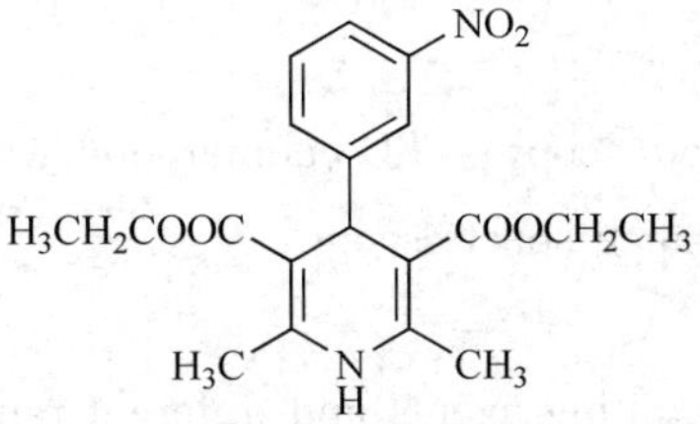

The product is a yellow crystal of powder, mp. 162-164℃, no moisture absorption, dissolved easily in acetone, dichloromethane, chloroform, dissolved in ethyl acetate. It dissolved slightly in methanol and ethanol, insolve in water.

The synthetic route is as follows:

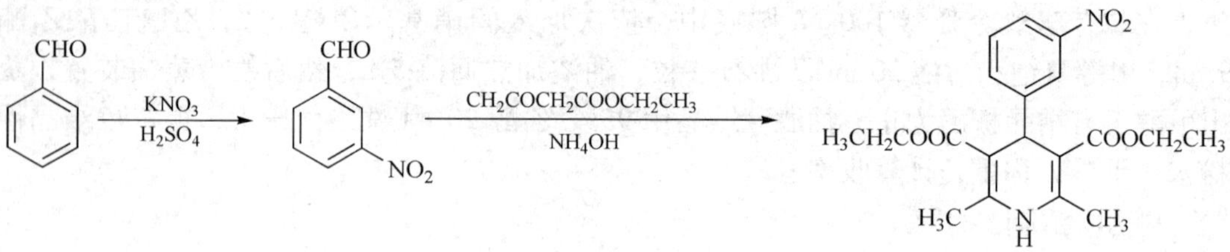

Experiment method

1. Nitrition

11 g of potassium nitrate is dissolved in 40ml of concentrated sulfuric acid, and then is put into a 250 ml three-necked flask equipped with a dropping funnel, a stirrer, a thermometer and immersed in an ice-salt bath. When the temperature of the solution reaches below 0℃, 10 g of benzaldehyde is added from dropping funnel slowly with vigorous stirring (60-90minutes), the temperature is required in 0-2℃ in this course. When the addition is finished, the mixture is stirred at 0-5℃ for 90 minutes by means of the ice-salt bath. The reaction mixture is then poured carefully into 200 ml of ice-water following stirring, and then separates out a yellow solid, filtered off. The filter cake is grinded into a powder in a mortar, and then 20 ml of 5% of sodium carbonate (1g/20 ml) is added. it continues to grind for 5 minutes, filtered off, the filter cake is ished with ice-water about 7-8 times, pressed to dry, *m*-nitrobenzaldehyde is obtained, air-dry (mp. 56-58℃), the yield is calculated.

2. Cyclization

5 g of *m*-nitro benzaldehyde, 9 ml of acetacetic ether, 30 ml of saturated solution of methanol, ammonia and a grain of zeolite are added into a 100 ml of round-bottomed flask equipped with a reflux condenser, the flask is heated and refluxed in an oil-bath for 5 h, and then distill methanol until crystal getten, filter off, the filter cake is ished with 20 ml of 95% of ethanol, pressed to dry and then yellow crystal is obtained, dry, weigh, calculate the yield.

3. Refinement

The crude product is recrystallized from 95% ethyl alcohol (5 ml/g), dry, measure mp. Weigh the product and calculate the yield.

4. Identification

① Infrared absorption spectroscopy; TLC counterpoint with standard substance.

② Nuclear magnetic resonance spectroscopy.

Notes:

1. Conclude the kinds of nitrating agents and different ranges of applications according to what you have learned.

2. Try to explain the mechanism of the cyclization reation.

实验十五 氯霉素（Chloramphenicol）的合成

【目的要求】

1. 熟悉溴化、Delepine 反应、乙酰化、羟甲基化、Meerwein－Ponndorf－Verley 羰基还原、水解、拆分、二氯乙酰化等反应的原理。

2. 掌握各步反应的基本操作和终点的控制。

3. 熟悉氯霉素及其中间体的立体化学。

4. 了解播种结晶法拆分外消旋体的原理，熟悉操作过程。

5. 掌握利用旋光仪测定光学异构体质量的方法。

【实验原理】

氯霉素的化学名为（1*R*,2*R*)-(－)-1-对硝基苯基-2-二氯乙酰胺基-1,3-丙二醇，(1*R*,2*R*) -(－)-*p*-nitropHenyl-2-dichloroacetamido-1,3-propanediol。氯霉素分子中有 2 个手性碳原子，有 4 个旋光异构体。化学结构式为：

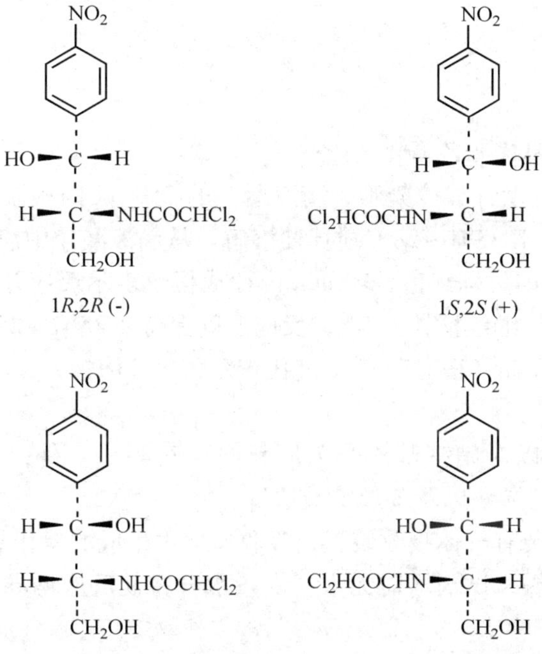

1*R*,2*R* (-)　　1*S*,2*S* (+)

1*S*,2*R* (-)　　1*R*,2*S* (+)

上面 4 个异构体中仅 1*R*,2*R*(－)〔或 D(－)苏阿糖型〕有抗菌活性，为临床使用的氯霉素。

氯霉素为白色或微黄色的针状、长片状结晶或结晶性粉末，味苦。mp. 149℃～153℃。易溶于甲醇、乙醇、丙酮或丙二醇中，微溶于水。比旋度 $[\alpha]^{25}$ －25. 5°（乙酸乙酯）；$[\alpha]_D^{25}$ ＋18. 5°～21. 5°（无水乙醇）。

合成路线如下：

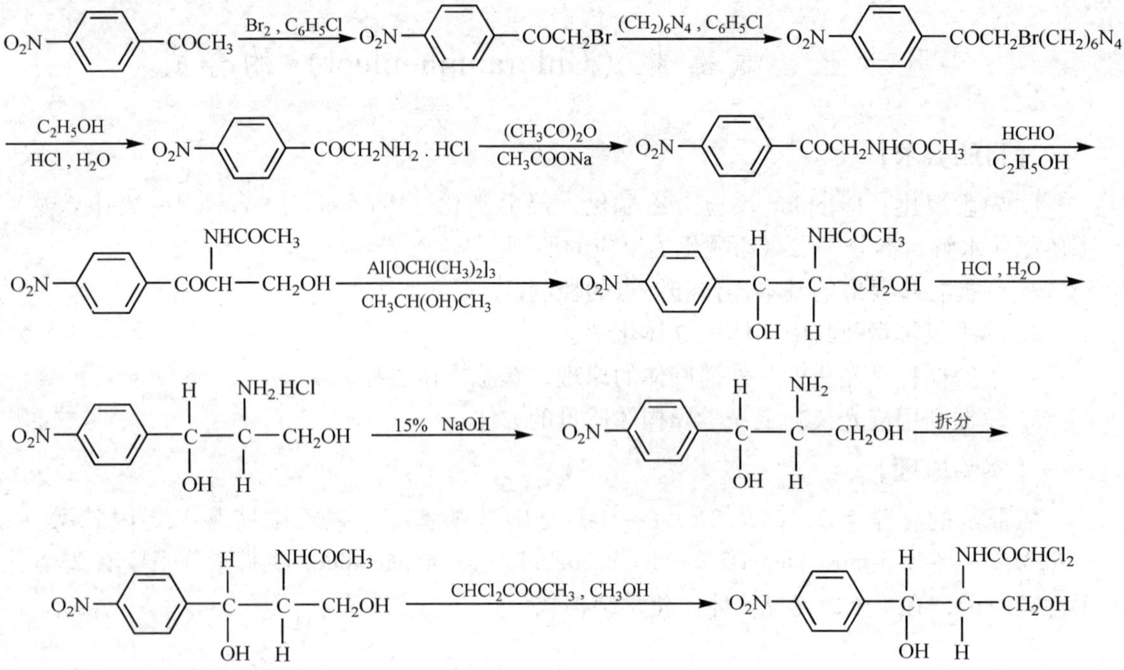

【实验方法】

（一）对硝基α-溴代苯乙酮的制备

在装有搅拌器、温度计、冷凝管、滴液漏斗的250 ml四颈瓶中，加入对硝基苯乙酮10 g，氯苯75 ml，于25℃～28℃搅拌使溶解。从滴液漏斗中滴加溴9.7 g。首先滴加溴2～3滴，反应液即呈棕红色，10 min内褪成橙色表示反应开始；继续滴加剩余的溴，约1～1.5 h加完，继续搅拌1.5 h，反应温度保持在25℃～28℃。反应完毕，水泵减压抽去溴化氢约30 min，得对硝基α-溴代苯乙酮氯苯溶液，备用。

[注释]

1. 制备氯霉素除以对硝基苯乙酮为原料的（对酮法）外，还有成肟法、苯乙烯法、肉桂醇法、溴苯乙烯法以及苯丝氨酸法等。

2. 冷凝管口上端装有气体吸收装置，吸收反应中生成的溴化氢。

3. 所用仪器应干燥，试剂均需无水。少量水分将使反应诱导期延长，较多水分甚至导致反应不能进行。

4. 若滴加溴后较长时间不反应，可适当提高温度，但不能超过50℃，当反应开始后要立即降低到规定温度。

5. 滴加溴的速度不宜太快，滴加速度太快及反应温度过高，不仅使溴积聚易逸出，而且还导致二溴化合物的生成。

6. 溴化氢应尽可能除去，以免下步消耗六亚甲基四胺。

[思考题]

1. 溴化反应开始时有一段诱导期，使用溴化反应机理说明原因。操作上如何缩短诱导期？

2. 本溴化反应不能遇铁，铁的存在对反应有何影响？

（二）对硝基 α-溴化苯乙酮六亚甲基四胺盐的制备

在装有搅拌器、温度计的 250 ml 三颈瓶中，依次加入上步制备好的对硝基 α-溴代苯乙酮和氯苯 20 ml，冷却至 15℃以下，在搅拌下加入六亚甲基四胺（乌洛托品）粉末 8.5 g，温度控制在 28℃以下，加毕，加热至 35℃～36℃，保温反应 1 h，测定终点。如反应已到终点，继续在 35℃～36℃反应 20 min，即得对硝基 α-溴代苯乙酮六亚甲基四胺盐（简称成盐物），然后冷至 16℃～18℃，备用。

[注释]

1. 此反应需无水条件，所用仪器及原料需经干燥，若有水分带入，易导致产物分解，生成胶状物。

2. 反应终点测定：取反应液少许，过滤，取滤液 1 ml，加入等量 4% 六亚甲基四胺三氯甲烷溶液，温热片刻，如不呈混浊，表示反应已经完全。

3. 对硝基 α-溴代苯乙酮六亚甲基四胺盐在空气中及干燥时极易分解，因此制成的复盐应立即进行下步反应，不宜超过 12 h。

4. 复盐成品：mp. 118℃～120℃（分解）。

[思考题]

1. 对硝基-α-溴代苯乙酮与六亚甲基四胺生成的复盐性质如何？

2. 成盐反应终点如何控制？根据是什么？

（三）对硝基-α-氨基苯乙酮盐酸盐的制备

在上步制备的成盐物氯苯溶液中加入精制食盐 3 g，浓盐酸 17.2 ml，冷至 6℃～12℃，搅拌 3～5 min，使成盐物呈颗粒状，待氯苯溶液澄清分层，分出氯苯。立即加入乙醇 37.7 ml，搅拌，加热，0.5 h 后升温到 32℃～35℃，保温反应 5 h。冷至 5℃以下，过滤，滤饼转移到烧杯中加水 19 ml，在 32℃～36℃搅拌 30 min，再冷至 －2℃，过滤，用预冷到 2℃～3℃的 6 ml 乙醇洗涤，抽干，得对硝基-α-氨基苯乙酮盐酸盐（简称水解物），mp. 250℃（分解），备用。

[注释]

1. 对硝基-α-溴代苯乙酮与六亚甲基四胺（乌洛托品）反应生成季铵盐，然后在酸性条件下水解成对硝基-α-氨基苯乙酮盐酸盐。该反应称 Delepine 反应。

2. 加入精盐在于减小对硝基-α-氨基苯乙酮盐酸盐的溶解度。

3. 成盐物水解要保持足够的酸度，所以与盐酸的摩尔比应在 3 以上。用量不仅导致生成醛等副反应（Sommolet 反应），而且对硝基-α-氨基苯乙酮游离碱本身亦不稳定，可发生双分子缩合，然后在空气中氧化成紫红色吡嗪化合物。此外，为保持水解液有足够酸度，应先加盐酸后加乙醇，以免生成醛等副反应。

4. 温度过高也易发生副反应，增加醛等副产物的生成。

[思考题]

1. 本实验中 Delepine 反应水解时为什么一定要先加盐酸后加乙醇，如果次序颠倒，结果会怎样？

2. 对硝基-α-氨基苯乙酮盐酸盐是强酸弱碱生成的盐，反应需保持足够的酸度，如果酸度不足对反应有何影响?

(四) 对硝基-α-乙酰胺基苯乙酮的制备

在装有搅拌器、回流冷凝器、温度计和滴液漏斗的 250 ml 四颈瓶中，放入上步制得的水解物及水 20 ml，搅拌均匀后冷至 0℃ ~5℃。在搅拌下加入醋酐 9 ml。另取 40% 的醋酸钠溶液 29 ml，用滴液漏斗在 30 min 内滴入反应液中，滴加时反应温度不超过 15℃。滴毕，升温到 14℃ ~15℃，搅拌 1 h（反应液始终保持在 pH 3.5 ~4.5），再补加醋酐 1ml，搅拌 10 min，测定终点。如反应已完全，立即过滤，滤饼用冰水搅成糊状，过滤，用饱和碳酸氢钠溶液中和至 pH 7.2 ~7.5，抽滤，再用冰水洗至中性，抽干，得淡黄色结晶（简称乙酰化物），mp. 161℃ ~163℃。

[注释]

1. 该反应需在酸性条件下（pH 3.5 ~4.5）进行，因此必须先加醋酐，后加醋酸钠溶液，次序不能颠倒。

2. 反应终点测定：取反应液少许，加入 $NaHCO_3$ 中和至碱性，于 40℃ ~45℃ 温热 30 min，不应呈红色。若反应未达终点，可补加适量的醋酐和醋酸钠继续酰化。

3. 乙酰化物遇光易变红色，应避光保存。

[思考题]

1. 乙酰化反应为什么要先加醋酐后加醋酸钠溶液，次序不能颠倒 ?

2. 乙酰化反应终点怎样控制，根据是什么?

(五) 对硝基-α-乙酰胺基-β-羟基苯丙酮的制备

在装有搅拌器、回流冷凝管、温度计的 250 ml 三颈瓶中，投入乙酰化物及乙醇 15 ml，甲醛 4.3 ml，搅拌均匀后用少量 $NaHCO_3$ 饱和溶液调 pH 7.2 ~7.5。搅拌下缓慢升温，大约 40 min 达到 32℃ ~35℃，再继续升温至 36℃ ~37℃，直到反应完全。迅速冷却至 0℃，过滤，用 25 ml 冰水分次洗涤，抽滤，干燥得对硝基-α-乙酰胺基-β-羟基苯丙酮（简称缩合物），mp. 166℃ ~167℃。

[注释]

1. 本反应碱性催化的 pH 值不宜太高，pH 7.2 ~7.5 较适宜。pH 过低反应不易进行，pH 大于 7.8 时有可能与两分子甲醛形成双缩合物。甲醛的用量对反应也有一定影响，如甲醛过量太多，亦有利于双缩合物的形成；用量过少，可导致一分子甲醛与两分子乙酰化物缩合。

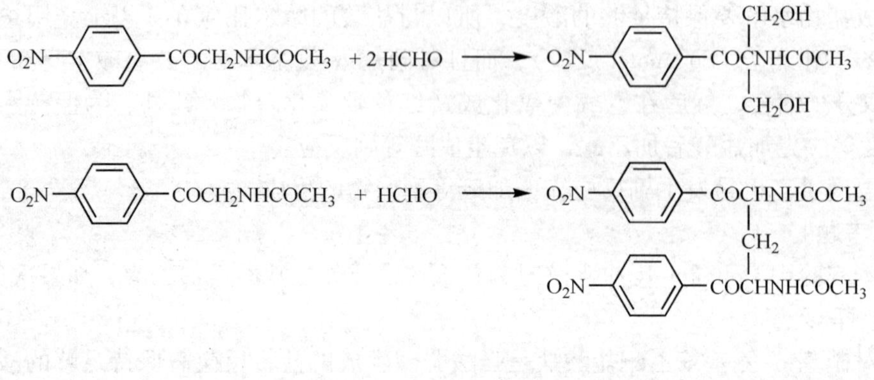

为了减少上述副反应，甲醛用量控制在过量40%左右（摩尔比约为1∶1.4）为宜。

2. 反应温度过高也有双缩合物生成，甚至导致产物脱水形成烯烃。

3. 反应终点测定：用玻棒蘸取少许反应液于载玻片上，加水1滴稀释后置显微镜下观察，如仅有羟甲基化合物的方晶而找不到乙酰化物的针晶，即为反应终点（约需3 h）。

[思考题]

1. 影响羟甲基化反应的因素有哪些？如何控制？

2. 羟甲基化反应为何选用$NaHCO_3$作为碱催化剂？能否用NaOH，为什么？

3. 羟甲基化反应终点如何控制？

（六）异丙醇铝的制备

在装有搅拌器、回流冷凝管、温度计的三颈瓶中依次投入剪碎的铝片2.7 g，无水异丙醇63 ml和无水三氯化铝0.3 g。在油浴上回流加热至铝片全部溶解，冷却到室温，备用。

[注释]

1. 所用仪器、试剂均应干燥无水。

2. 回流开始要密切注意反应情况，如反应太剧烈，需撤去油浴，必要时采取适当降温措施。

3. 如果无水异丙醇、无水三氯化铝质量好，铝片剪得较细，反应很快进行，约需1～2 h，即可完成。

（七）DL-苏阿糖型-1-对硝基苯基-2-氨基-1,3-丙二醇的制备

在上步制备异丙醇铝的三颈瓶中加入无水三氯化铝1.35 g，加热到44℃～46℃，搅拌30 min。降温到30℃，加入缩合物10 g。然后缓慢加热，约30 min内升温到58℃～60℃，继续反应4 h。冷却到10℃以下，滴加浓盐酸70 ml。滴毕，加热到70℃～75℃，水解2 h（最后0.5 h加入活性炭脱色），趁热过滤，滤液冷至5℃以下，放置1 h。过滤析出的固体，用少量20%盐酸（预冷至5℃以下）8 ml洗涤。然后将固体溶于12 ml水中，加热到45℃，滴加15% NaOH溶液到pH 6.5～7.6。过滤，滤液再用15% NaOH调节到pH 8.4～9.3，冷却至5℃以下，放置1 h。抽滤，用少量冰水洗涤，干燥，得DL-苏阿糖型-1-对硝基苯基-2-氨基-1,3-丙二醇（DL-氨基物），mp. 143℃～145℃。

[注释]

1. 滴加浓盐酸时温度迅速上升，注意控制温度不超过50℃。滴加浓盐酸促使乙酰化物水解，脱乙酰基，生成DL-氨基物盐酸盐，反应液中盐酸浓度大致在20%以上，此时$Al(OH)_3$形成了可溶性的$AlCl_3$-HCl复合物，而DL-氨基物盐酸盐在50℃以下溶解度小，过滤除去铝盐。

2. 用20% 盐酸洗涤的目的是除去附着在沉淀上的铝盐。

3. 用15% NaOH 溶液调节反应液到 pH 6.5 ~ 7.6，可以使残留的铝盐转变成 Al（OH）$_3$絮状沉淀过滤除去。

4. 还原后所得产物除 DL-苏阿糖型异构体外，尚有少量 DL-赤藓糖型异构体存在。由于后者的碱性较前者强，且含量少，在 pH 8.4 ~9.3 时，DL-苏阿糖型异构体游离析出，而 DL-赤藓糖型异构体仍留在母液中而分离。

［思考题］

1. 制备异丙醇铝的关键有哪些？

2. Meerwein-Ponndorf-Verley 还原反应中加入少量 $AlCl_3$有何用？

3. 试解释异丙醇铝-异丙醇还原 DL-对硝基-α-乙酰胺基-β-羟基苯丙酮主要生成 DL-苏阿糖型氨基物的理由。

4. 还原产物 1-对硝基苯基-2-乙酰氨基-1,3-丙二醇水解脱乙酰基，为什么用 HCl 而不用 NaOH 水解？水解后产物为什么用 20 % 盐酸洗涤？

5. “氨基醇”盐酸盐碱化时为什么要二次碱化？

（八）D-(－)-1-对硝基苯基-α-氨基-1,3-丙二醇的制备

1. 拆分

在装有搅拌器、温度计的 250 ml 三颈瓶中投入 DL-氨基物 5.3 g，L-氨基物2.1 g，DL-氨基物盐酸盐 16.5 g 和蒸馏水 78 ml。搅拌，水浴加热，保持温度在 61℃ ~63℃反应约 20 min，使固体全部溶解。然后缓慢自然冷却至 45℃，开始析出结晶。再在 70 min内缓慢冷却至 29℃ ~30℃，迅速抽滤，用热蒸馏水 3 ml（70℃）洗涤，抽干，干燥，得微黄色结晶（粗 L-氨基物），mp. 157℃ ~159℃。滤液中再加入 DL-氨基物 4.2 g，按上法重复操作，得粗 D-氨基物。

2. 精制

在 100 ml 烧杯中加入 D-或 L-氨基物 4.5 g，1 mol / L 稀盐酸 25 ml。加热到 30℃ ~35℃使溶解，加活性炭脱色，趁热过滤。滤液用 15% NaOH 溶液调至 pH 9.3，析出结晶。再在 30℃ ~35℃保温 10 min，抽滤，用蒸馏水洗至中性，抽干，干燥，得白色结晶，mp. 160℃ ~162℃。

3. 旋光测定

取本品 2.4 g，精密称定，置 100 ml 容器中加 1 mol / L 盐酸（不需标定）至刻度，按照旋光度测定法测定（《中国药典》1995 版二部附录 38 页），应为（＋)/(－) 1.36° ~ （＋)/(－) 1.40°。

根据旋光度计算：含量（%）$=(100\times\alpha)/(2\times2.4\times29.5)\times100\%$

其中：α = 旋光度

29.5 = 换算系数

2 = 管长为 2 dm

2.4 = 样品的百分浓度

［注释］

1. DL-氨基物盐酸盐的制备：在 250 ml 烧杯中放置 DL-氨基物 30 g，搅拌下加入 20% 盐酸 39 ml（浓盐酸 22 ml，水 17 ml）。加毕，置水浴中加热至完全溶解，放置，自然冷却，当有固体析出时不断缓慢搅拌，以免结块。最后冷至 5℃，放置 1 h，过滤，滤饼用 95% 乙醇洗涤，干燥，即得 DL-氨基物盐酸盐。

2. 固体必须全溶，否则结晶提前析出。

3. 严格控制降温速度，仔细观察初析点和全析点，正常情况下初析点为45℃ ~47℃。

（九）氯霉素的制备

在装有搅拌器、回流冷凝器、温度计的 100 ml 三颈瓶中，加入 D-氨基物 4.5 g，甲醇 10 ml 和二氯乙酸甲酯 3 ml。在 60℃ ~65℃搅拌反应 1 h，随后加入活性炭 0.2 g，保温脱色 3 min，趁热过滤，向滤液中滴加蒸馏水（每分钟约 1ml 的速度滴加）至有少量结晶析出时停止加水，稍停片刻，继续加入剩余蒸馏水（共 33 ml）。冷至室温，放置 30 min，抽滤，滤饼用 4 ml 蒸馏水洗涤，抽干，105℃干燥，即得氯霉素，mp. 149.5℃ ~153℃。

［注释］

1. 反应必须在无水条件下进行，有水存在时，二氯乙酸甲酯水解成二氯乙酸，与氨基物成盐，影响反应的进行。

2. 二氯乙酰化除用二氯乙酸甲酯作为酰化剂外，二氯乙酸酐、二氯乙酸胺、二氯乙酰氯均可作酰化剂，但用二氯乙酸甲酯成本低，酰化收率高。

3. 二氯乙酸甲酯的质量直接影响产品的质量，如有一氯或三氯乙酸甲酯存在，同样能与氨基物发生酰化反应，形成的副产物带入产品，致使熔点偏低。

4. 二氯乙酸甲酯的用量略多于理论量，以弥补因少量水分水解的损失，保证反应完全。

［思考题］

1. 二氯乙酰化反应除用二氯乙酸甲酯外，还可用哪些试剂，生产上为何采用二氯乙酸甲酯？

2. 二氯乙酸甲酯的质量和用量对产物有何影响？

3. 试对我国生产氯霉素的合成路线和其他合成路线作一评价。

（十）结构确证

1. 红外吸收光谱法、标准物 TLC 对照法。

2. 核磁共振光谱法。

Experiment 15 Synthesis of Chloramphenicol

Purpose

1. To have an intimate knowledge of cylite, Delepine, acetylate, hydroxymethylation, Meerwein-Ponndorf-Verley carbonyl reduction, hydrolization, split and dichloro acetylate reaction.

2. To grasp the basic manipulate of each step and the control of end point.

3. To have an intimate knowledge of the stereochemistry of chloramphenicol and its pivotal intermediate.

4. To comprehend the axiom of splitting racemic body by inoc crystal method.

5. To grasp the method of determining the quality of optics isomer by polarimeter.

Mechanism

The chemical name of chloramphenicol is (1*R*,2*R*)-(−)-*p*-nitrophenyl-2-dichloroacetamido-1,3-propanediol. There are two chiral centers in chloramphenicol molecule. It has four optical isomers. The chemical structural formula is below:

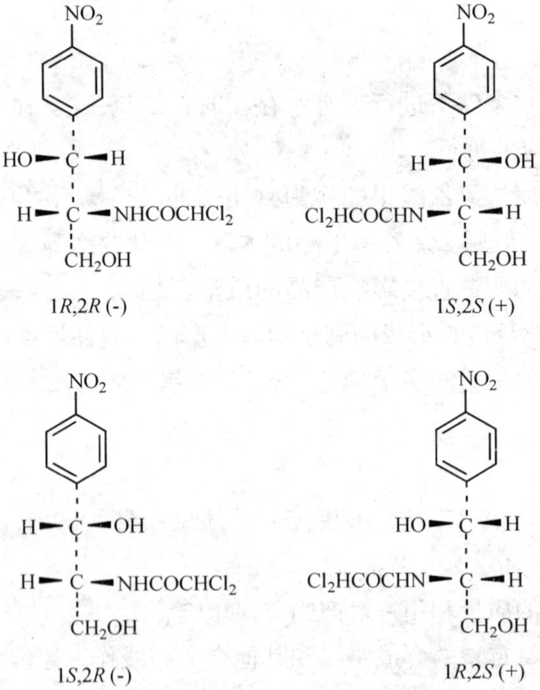

Only 1*R*,2*R*(−) has antibacterial activity. It is used in clinic.

Chloramphenicol is a white or yellowish needle dolicho-lamellar crystal or crystallinity powder, bitter in taste. Mp.: 149-153℃ (dec.), which is slightly soluble in water, but dissoluble in methanol, acetone, ethanol and propylene glycol. Specific optical rotation $[\alpha]^{25}$ −25.5° (acetic ether); $[\alpha]_D^{25}$ +18.5°-21.5° (absolute alcohol).

Route:

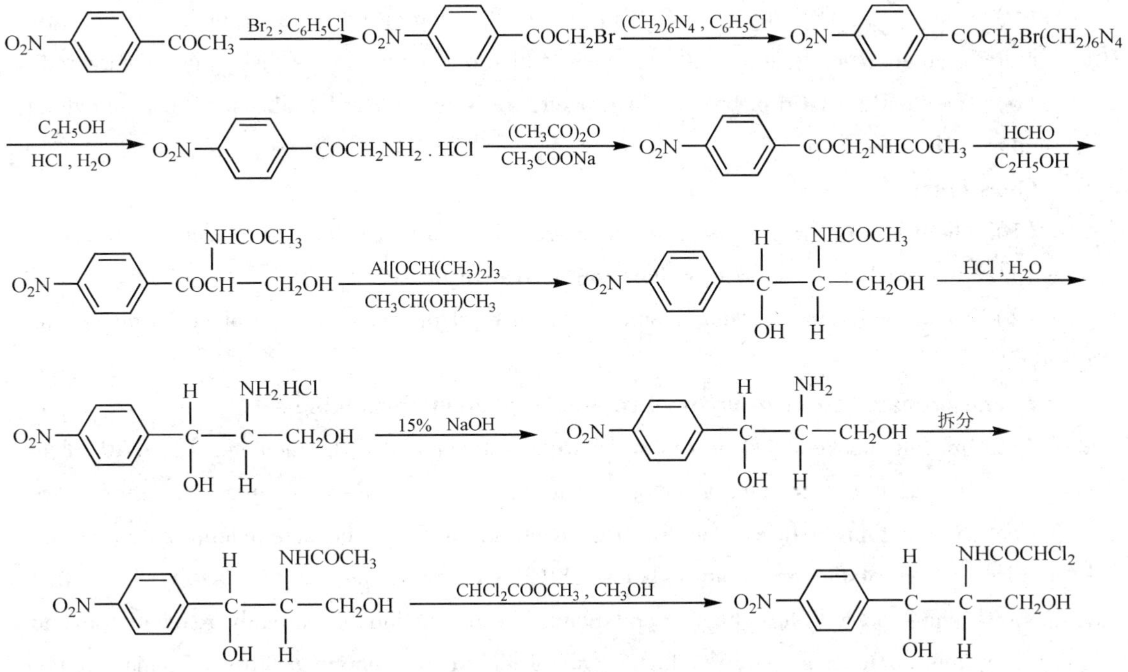

Experiment method

1. The preparation of antinitro-α-bromacetophenone

A 250ml four-necked flask is equipped with a stirrer, a thermometer, a condensation tube and a dropping funnel. 10 g of antinitro-acetophenone, 75 ml of chlorobenzene is added to the flask. Stir this solution to resolve the solid at 25-28℃. Drop 9. 7 g of bromine to the mixture by the dropping funnel. First, add 2-3 drops of bromine to the mixture. The liquid offers Bronish red color. The reaction starts when it change to orange in 10 min, continue to add the surplus bromine in about 1-1. 5 hour. Stir it for 1. 5 hours. The temperature is keeped about 25℃-28℃. After that, draw bromide hydrogen by water pump deboost for 30 mins. The *p*-nitro-α-bromacetophenone will be abtioned.

Notes:

(1) Besides using *p*-nitroacetophenone as stock, there are still some left oxim method, benzene vinyl method, cinnamic alcohol method, brombenzene vinyl method and serine method.

(2) Gas absorption plant is equipped on the top of the condensation tube to the absorb bromide hydrogen which is producted in this reaction.

(3) All the equipment should be dried. The agent should be anhydrous. Small amounts of water will prolong the derivative phase. Hyperhydration even can prevent the reaction from carrying out.

(4) If the reaction don't start after the addition of bromine, we can raise the temperature. Keep the temperature below 50℃. It should be cut down to defined temperature when the

reaction starts.

(5) Control the dropping rate of bromide, swift dropping rate and hyperpyrexia not only lead bromine to accumulate and emit, but also induce the production of disbromine compound.

(6) We should get rid of bromide hydrogen, in order to avoid analosising hexamethylene tetramine in the next step.

Questions:

(1) There is a derivative phase when the reaction starts. Explain the reason using bromination reaction mechanism. How to reduce the derivative phase?

(2) This bromination reaction should not meet Fe. How does the exist of Fe influence this reaction?

2. The preparation of *p*-nitro-α-brom acetophenone hexamine salt

A 250ml four-necked flask is equipped with a stirrer and a thermometer. Place 20 ml of chlorobenzene and *p*-nitro-α-bromacetophenone which had been obtained in the above step. Cool the reaction mixture to below 15℃. Then add 8.5 g of hexamethylene tetramine and keep stirring. Control the temperature below 28℃. After that, heat it to 35-36℃. Keep that temperature for 1 hour. Determine the end point. If the reaction has already reached the end point, continue to react at 35-36℃ for 20 min. Then we will obtain *p*-nitro-α-bromacetophenone hexamine salt. Cool it to 16-18℃.

Notes:

(1) This reaction needs anhydrous condition. The equipment and mat should be dried. If some water is taken in, it is easy to result in the decomposition of product and the production of dope.

(2) Determine the end point of the reaction: take a bit of reaction juice, filter it. Take 1ml of filtrate, add 1ml of 4% hexamethylene tetramine, thermy and heat for a moment. If it does not offer cloudiness, demonstrate the reaction has been completely.

(3) *p*-nitro-α-brom acetophenone hexamine salt is easy to decompose when it is arescent or in the air. So the compound salt which is producted should be used in the next step immediately.

(4) Compound salt finished product: mp. 118-120℃ (decompose).

Questions:

(1) What is the character of the compound salt which the p-nitro-α-bromacetophenone and hexamethylene tetramine formned?

(2) How to control the end point of salt forming reaction? What is the evidence?

3. The preparation of *p*-nitro-α-aminoacetophenone muriate

Add 3 g of depurate common salt and 17.2 ml of concentrated hydrochloric acid into the solution which is prepared in the above step. Cool the mixture to 6-12℃. Stir it for 3-5min. When the chlorobenzene solution clear and demix, diverge chlorobenzene out. Add 37.7 ml of alcohol immediately. Stir and heat it. The temperature rises to 32-35℃ after 0.5

hour. Keep the temperature for about 5 hours. Cool it to below 5℃ and filter it. Transfer the filter cake to a beaker and add 19 ml of water. Stir it at 32-36℃ for 30 mins. Cool it to -2℃ and filter it. Ish it with 6ml of alcohol which had been cooled to 2-3℃. Sucking filter the mixture until it is dry. *p*-nitro-α-aminoacetophenone muriate will be obtained. Mp. 250℃

Notes:

(1) *p*-nitro-α-aminoacetophenone and hexamethylene tetramine react and form quaternary ammonium salt. Then the quaternary ammonium salt hydrolyzes to *p*-nitro-α-aminoacetophenone muriate. This reaction is named Delepine reaction.

(2) The reason for addition of refined salt is to reduce the dissolubility of *p*-nitro-α-aminoacetophenone muriate.

(3) The hydrolization of salification matter should be keeped above pH 3. Dosage can result in Sommolet reaction. *p*-nitro-α-aminoacetophenone free alkali is instability. It can condense between two molecules. Then it will be oxidized and product prunosus pyrazine compound. In addition, we should add hydrochloric acid before adding ethanol to keep the digest having enough acescence and avoid adverse reaction.

(4) Hyperpyrexia may result in adverse reaction and increase the production of aldehyde.

Questions:

(1) What is the reason for adding chlorhydric acid before adding ethanol? If we change the turn, what is the result will be?

(2) *p*-nitro-α-aminoacetophenone muriate is the salt which is made from the reaction of strong acid and weak base. The reaction should keep enough acidity. If acescence is not enough, what influence will be?

4. The preparation of *p*-nitro-α-acetamidoacetophenone

A 250ml four-necked flask is equipped with a stirrer, a thermometer, a condensation tube and a dropping funnel. Place 20ml of water and hydrolyzate which had been prepared in the above step. Stir this solution and cool it to 0-5℃. Add 9 ml of acetic anhydride and keep stirring. Take 29 ml of 40% sodium acetate solution. Drop it to the mixture by the dropping funnel in 30 mins and keep the internal temperature below 15℃. After that, heat it to 14-15℃. Stir it for 1 hour(Keep the PH of the mixture at 3. 5-4. 5). Add 1 ml of acetic anhydride and stir it for 10 mins. Determine the end point. If the reaction has been completed, filter it immediately. Stir the filter cake to pasty with ice-water. Filter it and counteract it to pH 7. 2-7. 5 with equilibrium sodium bicarbonate solution. Sucking filter it and ish it to neutrality with ice-water. Sucking filter the mixture until it is dry. An amber crystal will be obtained (call for short acetylate), mp: 161-163℃.

Note:

(1) The reaction should be carried out under acidity condition (pH 3. 5-4. 5) . So we should add acetic anhydride before adding sodium acetate solution. The order should not be re-

versed.

(2) Determine the end point: take a little of reaction liquid, add sodium bicarbonate to counteract it to alkalinity. Heat it for 30 mins at 40-45℃. It should not offer red. If the reaction has not reached the end point, we can add acetic anhydride and natrium aceticum to make the acylation continue.

(3) When the acetylate meets light, it is easy to change red. We should keep it far from light.

Questions:

(1) What is the reason for adding acetic anhydride before adding sodium acetate solution?

(2) How to control the end point of acetylate reaction? What is the evidence?

5. The reparation of *p*-nitro-α-acetamido-β-hydroxylcoumadin

A 250ml four-necked flask is equipped with a stirrer, a thermometer, a condensation tube and a dropping funnel. Place 15 ml of acetylate, 4. 3 ml of formaldehyde and 15 ml of ethanol. Dilute the mixture and add sodium bicarbonate saturated solution to adjust the pH to 7. 2-7. 5. Heat the solution to 32-35℃ for about 40 mins and keep stirring. Continue to heat it to 36-37℃ until the reaction has been completely. Cool it to 0℃. Filter it and ish it with ice-water. Sucking filter and dry it. *p*-nitro-α-acetamido-β-hydroxylcoumadin will be obtained. mp. 166-167℃.

Notes:

(1) Alky catalytic pH is not suitable in high in this procedure, pH 7. 2-7. 5 is most suitable. The reaction will not be easy to carry out in low pH, it may form couple condensation compound with two formaldehyde molecule.

The dosage of formaldehyde has some effects to the reaction, too. For example if it is too much, also may be profit to form couple condensation compound; and if it is too little, may lead to one molecular formaldehyde condensing with two molecular acetylate.

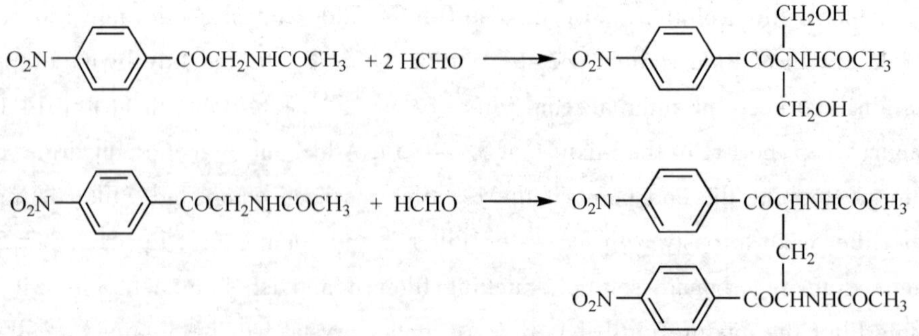

In order to reduce adverse reaction above-mentioned, the dosage of formaldehyde should be controled about overdose 40% (molar ratio 1 : 1. 4 or so).

(2) Hyperpyrexia may also have coupled condensation compound generated, even lead

to the product being dehydrated to alkenes.

(3) The determination of the terminal of the reaction :

Dip a little reaction liquid on glass slide, imbibe one drop to dilute then to observe under microscope. If only find cubic crystal of hydroxymethyl compound and haven't found acicular crystal of acetylate, it is the terminal of the reaction (about 3h) .

Questions:

(1) What are the facts that effect hydroxymethlation reaction? How to control it?

(2) Why to choose $NaHCO_3$ as base catalyst in hydroxymethylation reaction. What about NaOH, Why ?

(3) How to control the termination of the hydroxymethylation reaction?

6. The preparation of Aluminum isopropanol

In a three-necked bottle equipped with an agitator, a reflux condensing tube, a thermometer, place smashed sheet 2.7 g of aluminum 63ml of anhydi-avanti and 0.3 g of anhy di-aluminium trichloride. Reflux on an oil bath to the all sheet aluminum to dissolve. Cool it to room temperature pre-emergency.

Notes:

(1) The equipments and agents should be both dryed.

(2) The information of the reaction must be watched closely when the reflux begins. If it is too severe, remove the oil bath. Some suitable measures to reduce the temperature should be taken in prorenate.

(3) If the quality of anhydrous isopropanol and aluminum chloride is good, and sheet aluminum is sliced thin, the reaction is very quick for 1-2 h.

7. The preparation of DL-threose-1-para Nitrophenyl-2-amino-1,3-propylene glycol

Place 1.35g of andydrons-aluminum trichloride into the three-necked bottle that last step is used in preparing aluminium isopropoxide, heat to 44-46℃, stir for 30 mins. Reduce to 30℃, add condensation compound 10g. Then heat slowly. Rise the temperature to 58-60℃ in about 30 mins, continue reacting for 4h. Cool to below 10℃, drop 70 ml of concentrated hydrochloric acid. Heat to 70-75℃, hydrolyzed for 2 h (throw into activated carbon for bleaching in the last 0.5h), filtering while it is hot. Cool filtrate to below 5℃, lay up 1h. Filter the separated solid, ished with a small quantity ice water, drying, obtain DL-threose-1-para Nitrophenyl-2-amino-1, 3-propylene glycol (DL-amid-substratum), mp. 143℃-145℃.

Note:

(1) The temperature will rise fast while dropwise concentrated hydrochlorid acid, pay attention to control the temperature below 50℃. Dropwise concentrated hydrochlorid acid in order to hydrolyze acetylate, to cast off ethanoyl, generate DL-amid-substratum muriaficus. The hydrochloride acid concentration of reaction liquid should be about above 20%, while, $Al(OH)_3$ has formed dissoluble $AlCl_3$-HCl complexes, and the dissolubility of DL-amid-sub-

stratum is little, get rid of aluminum salt by filtering.

(2) The purpose of ish with 20% hydrochlorid acid is to get rid of aluminum salt that accretes on the sediment.

(3) To adjust pH of reaction liquid to pH 6.5-7.6 with 15% NaOH solution, can change the aluminum salt to $Al(OH)_3$ flocculent and get rid of it.

(4) The product that gets from reduction beside isomeride of DL-threose, also has some isomeride DL-erythrose. The alky of later is stronger than the former, and the content is little, while the pH is 8.4-9.3, the isomeride of DL-threose isolated, and the isomeride of DL-erythrose still remains in mother liquid.

Questions:

(1) What is the key point of preparing AIP?

(2) What is the function of throwing a little of $AlCl_3$ into Meerwein-Ponndorf-Verley reduction reaction.

(3) Try to explain the reason that AIP-avantin reducts DL-para nitro-α-acetic amid-β-hydroxide radical coumadin, generates DL-threose amid sabstratum mainly.

(4) The reduction product 1-para-nitrophenyl-2-acetamido-1,3-propylene hydrolizated and get rid of acetyl group, why did hydrolization with HCl but not NaOH? Why ish the output of hydrolization with 20% hydrochloric acid?

(5) Why should be alkalified twice when "aminoalcohol" was alkalified by muriaficus?

8. The preparation of D-(-)-1-para nitrophenyl-α-amino-group-1, 3-propylene

(1) split Throw 5.3 g of DL-amino substratum, 2.1 g of L-amino substratum, 16.5g of DL-amino substratum muriaficus and distilled water into a 250ml three-necked bottle equipped with an agitator, a thermometer. Stir, to heat in water bath, keep the temperature at 61-63℃, react for about 20 mins, until all the solid is dissolved. Then naturally coolslowly to 45℃, begin to crystallize. Then slowly cool to 29-30℃ in 70 mins. Then sucking filtrate quickly. Ished with hot distilled water 3 ml (70℃), sucking filtrate to dry, obtain subtle yellow crystal (coarse L-amino substratum), mp. 157-159℃. Throw 4.2 g of DL-amino substratum into the filter liquor. Repetitive operation as before, obtain coarse D-amino substratum.

(2) Depuration Throw 4.5 g of D-or L-amino substratum, 25ml of 1mol/L dilute hydrochloric acid into a 100 ml beaker. Heat to 30-35℃ in order to dissolve. Put in activated carbon, filter while hot. adjust filter liquor to pH 9.3 with 15% NaOH solution, separates crystal. Then incubate in 30-35℃ for 10 mins, sucking filtration. Ished to neutral with distilled water. Filter it until it is dried. A white crystal will be obtained. mp. 160-162℃.

(3) Optical rotation determination Take 2.4 g of it, weigh it precisely, place into a 100 ml container and add 1 mol/L hydrochloric acid to reach the scale. Determine it according to optical rotation assay. It should be(+)/(-)1.36° ~ (+)/(-)1.40°.

Calculate according to optical rotation:

content% = $(100\times\alpha)/(2\times2.4\times29.5)\times100\%$

α = optical rotation

29.5 = conversion factor

2 = tube length is 2 dm

2.4 = the percentage concentration of essay

Notes:

(1) The preparation of DL-amid muriaficus: Place 30 g of DL-amid muriaficus into a 250 ml beaker. Add 39 ml of 20% chlorhydric acid and keep stirring (22 ml of concentrated hydrochloric acid and 17 ml of water). After that, heat it in a water bath until it dissolves completely. Lay it up and cool it. When the solid precipitates, stir it to avoid agglomerate. Cool it to 5℃, lay up for 1h, filtering, then ish it with 95% alcohol, dry, obtain DL-amino substratum hydrochlorid acid.

(2) All the solid must be dissolved, or the crystal will separate ahead of schedule.

(3) The speed of reducing temperature must be controlled strictly. Observe the time which the crystalization begins and is over. The normal temperature of the beginning is 45-47 ℃.

9. the preparation of amphemycin

Throw 4.5 g of D-amino substratum, 10ml of methanol, 3 ml of rysta bichloracetic acid into the 100 ml three-necked bottle equipped with an agitator, a reflux condenser, a thermometer. To stir and react for 1h at 60-65℃, then add 0.2 g of activated carbon, incubation bleach for 3min, to filter while hot, drop distilled water into the filter liquor(1ml per min). Stop dropping until some crystal begins to restallize. Stay for a moment, go on dropping the surplus distilled water (about 33 ml). Cool to room temperature, lay up for 30 min, sucking filtration, ish the filtration with 4 ml distilled water, draw to dry. Dry at 105℃, obtain amphemycin. mp. 149-153℃.

Notes:

(1) The reaction must be carried out in anhydrous condition, if water exists, methyl ester bichloracetic will hydrolyze to bichloracetic, salificate with amino substratum, influence the progress of the reaction.

(2) Besides using dichloromethyl acetate as acylating agent in dichloro acetylate reaction, we can also use dichloroacetic anhydride, dichloroacetic amine, dichloroacetyl chloride. But the cost is low and the acylation yield is high by using dichloromethyl acetate.

(3) The quality of dichloromethyl acetate directly influences the quality of product. If there is chloromethyl acetate or trichloromethyl acetate, the acylation reaction with amidont also can happen. The by-product which the reaction producted sneaks into product, resulting in the melting point lower.

(4) The practical dosage of dichloromethyl acetate exceedes theoretical dosage to retrieve the loss caused by the hydrolization of water and ensure the reaction completely.

Questions:

(1) Besides using dichloromethyl acetate in the dichloro acetylate reaction, what other agents we can use? Why do we use dichloromethyl acetate in production?

(2) How do the quality and dosage of the dichloromethyl acetate effect the production?

(3) Try to estimate the synthetic route of the product of chloramphenicol in our country and the others.

10. structure ascertainment

(1) Infrared absorption spectrum method, standard substance TLC confrontation method.

(2) Nuclear magentic resonance spectroscopy.

实验十六 地巴唑（Dibazole）的合成

【目的要求】

1. 熟悉合成杂环药物的方法。
2. 掌握脱水反应原理及操作技术。

【实验原理】

地巴唑为降压药，对血管平滑肌有直接松弛作用，使血压略有下降。可用于轻度的高血压和脑血管痉挛等。地巴唑化学名为α-苄基苯并咪唑盐酸盐，化学结构式为：

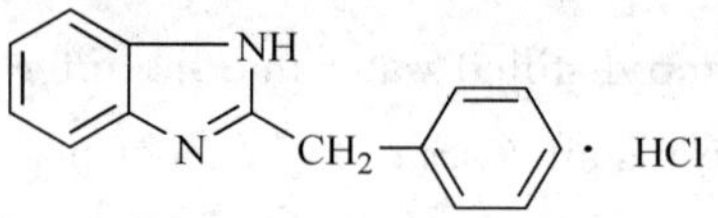

地巴唑为白色结晶性粉末，无臭。mp. 182℃ ~186℃，几乎不溶于三氯甲烷和苯，略溶于热水或乙醇。

合成路线如下：

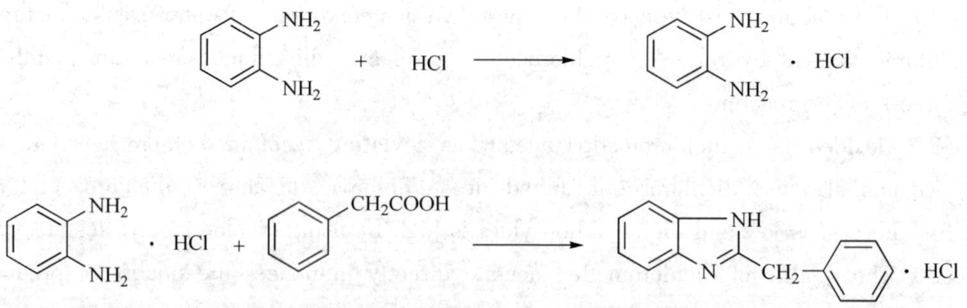

【实验方法】

（一）成盐

将浓盐酸11.2 ml稀释至17.4 ml，取其半量加入50 ml烧杯中，盖上表面皿，于石棉网上加热至近沸。一次加入邻苯二胺用玻璃棒搅拌，使固体溶解，然后加入余下的盐酸和活性炭1 g，搅匀，趁热抽滤。滤液冷却后，析出结晶，抽滤，结晶用少量乙醇洗3次，抽干，干燥，得白色或粉红色针状结晶，即为邻苯二胺单盐酸盐。测熔点，计算收率。

（二）环合

在装有搅拌器、温度计和蒸馏装置的60 ml三颈瓶中，加入苯乙酸适量（苯乙酸与邻苯二胺单盐酸盐的摩尔比为1.06∶1），沙浴加热，使内温达99℃～100℃。待苯乙酸熔化后，在搅拌下加入邻苯二胺单盐酸盐（将上一步产品全部投料）。升温至150℃开始脱水，然后慢慢升温，于160℃～240℃反应3 h（大部分时间控制在200℃左右）。反应结束后，使反应液冷却到150℃以下，趁热慢慢向反应液中加入4倍量的沸水（按邻苯二胺单盐酸盐计算），搅拌溶解，加活性炭脱色，趁热抽滤，将滤液立即转移到烧杯中，搅拌，冷却，结晶（防止结成大块）抽滤，结晶用少量水洗3次，得地巴唑盐基粗品。

（三）盐基的精制

取约为地巴唑盐基湿粗品5.5倍量的水，加入烧杯中，加热煮沸，投入地巴唑盐基粗品，加热溶解后，用10%氢氧化钠调节到pH 9，冷却，抽滤，结晶用少量蒸馏水洗至中性，抽干，即得地巴唑盐基精品。

（四）成盐

将地巴唑盐基湿品用1.5倍量蒸馏水调成糊状，加热，抽滤，结晶用盐酸调节pH 4～5，使完全溶解。加活性炭脱色，趁热抽滤，使滤液冷却，析出结晶，用蒸馏水洗3次，得地巴唑盐粗品。

（五）盐的精制

将地巴唑盐粗品用2倍量蒸馏水加热溶解，加活性炭脱色，趁热抽滤，滤液冷却，析出结晶。抽滤，用蒸馏水洗3次，抽干，干燥，测熔点，计算收率。

（六）结构确证

1. 红外吸收光谱法、标准物TLC对照法。

2. 核磁共振光谱法。

［注释］

1. 用盐酸溶解邻苯二胺时，温度不宜过高，约80℃～90℃即可，否则所生成的邻苯二胺单盐酸盐颜色变深。由于邻苯二胺单盐在水中溶解度较大，故所用仪器应尽量干燥。邻苯二胺单盐酸盐制好后，应先在空气中吹去大部分溶媒，然后再于红外灯下干燥。否则，产品长时间在红外灯下照射，易被氧化成浅红色。

2. 在环合反应过程中，气味较大，可将出气口导至水槽，温度上升速度视蒸出水的速度而定。开始由160℃逐渐升至200℃，较长时间维持在200℃左右，最后半小时升至240℃，但不得超过240℃，否则邻苯二胺被破坏，产生黑色树脂状物，产率明显下降。在加入沸水前，反应液须冷却到150℃以下，以防反应瓶破裂。

3. 在精制地巴唑盐基时，结晶用少量蒸馏水洗至中性的目的是洗去未反应的苯乙酸。

【思考题】

1. 在邻苯二胺单盐酸盐制备中，取半量盐酸加热近沸，此时为什么温度不宜过高？
2. 环合反应温度太高有何不利？为什么？
3. 试解释合成苯并咪唑环的环合反应机理？

Experiment 16 Synthesis of Dibazole

Purpose

1. To be familiar with the way of the synthesis of heterocyclic druggery.
2. To predominate the principle of dehydrate reaction and operation skill

Mechanism

Dibazole is a kind of antihypertensive drug, used in the action of straight slack of glabrate muscle of blood vessel, longitudinal high blood pressure, to drop the blood pressure.

Its chemical name is: α-phenylbenzimidazole hydrochloric acid salt. Its chemical structure is as follows:

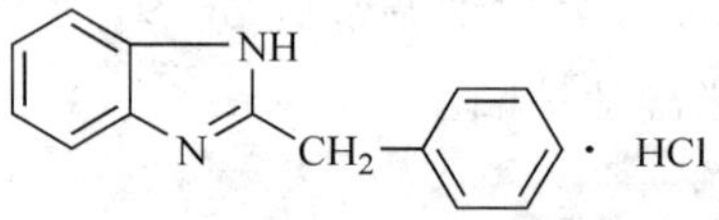

Dibazole is a white crystal powder, mp: 182-186℃, almost insolve in chloroform and benzene, dissolve in hot water or alcohol.

The synthetic route is as follows:

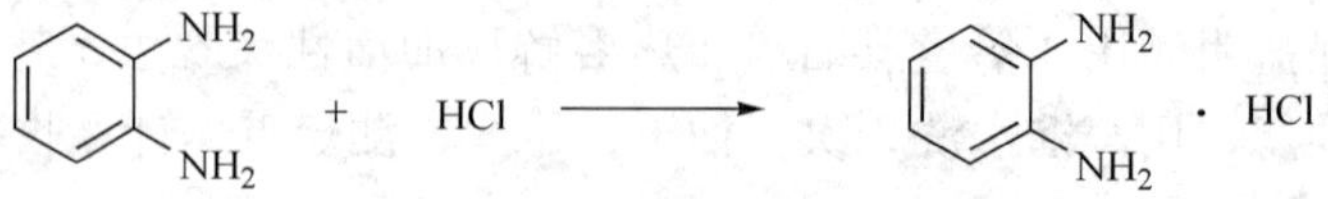

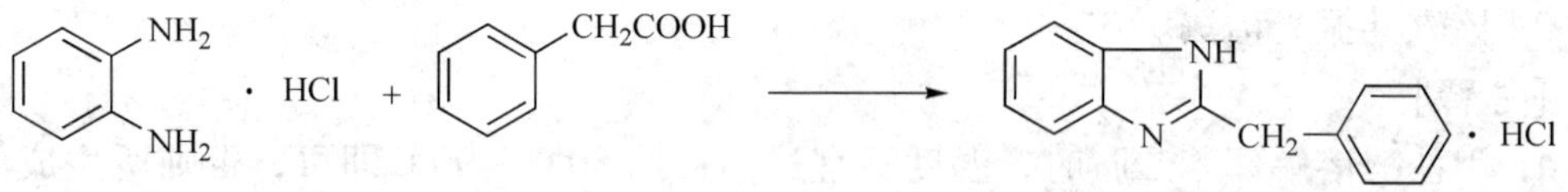

Experiment method

1. Being salt

11. 2ml of concentrated hydrochloric acid is diluted to 17. 4 ml, take a half of it into a 50 ml beaker, cover the watch glass on the beaker and heat up to almost boiling on an asbestos gauge. Portions of *o*-phenylendiamine are added into the beaker following stirring to make the solid dissolve, and then the other hydrochloric acid and active carbon are also added into it. Stir and filter out when the solution is hot, cool and filter out, the crystal is ished with alcohol three times, dry and get white or pink crystal of needles, detect mp, calculate the

yield.

2. Cyclization

Phenyl acetic acid (phenyl acetic acid: mono-salt hydrochloric acid *o*-phenylendiamine =1.06 : 1) is added into a 60ml three-necked flask equipped with a device of distillation, a stirrer, athermometer and immersed in asand-bath that makes the temperature at 99-100℃. When the phenyl acetic acid melts, mono-salt hydrochloric acid *o*-phenylendiamine is added into the flask following stirring, when the temperature is 150℃, the dehydration starts, and then the temperature raises slowly and reacts for 3h at 160-240℃ (mostly 200℃). When the reaction ends, the solution is cooled below 150℃, and four times of boiling water are added into the solution (according to mono-salt *o*-phenylendiamine), stir to dissolve and then the activated carbon is added, filter out when the solution is hot, the filtrate is moved into the beaker immediately, stir, cool, filter out the crystal and then ish it with a little water three times, and get the crude product.

3. Refinement

5.5 times of the crude of water are added into the beaker, heat up to boil, and then the crude is added into the beaker, heated up to dissolve, 10% sodium hydroxide is used to adjust pH to 9, cool, filter out, the crystal is ished by distilled water to neutrality, dry, and get the extraction.

4. Being salt

The wet product of salt-Dibazole is adjusted to be paste by 1.5 times of distilled water and then heated up, filtered, and the crystal is adjusted to pH 4-5 by hydrochloric acid to make it dissolved. The activated carbon is added and then filtered out when the solution is hot, the filtrate is cooled and get the crystals, the crystals are ished by the distilled water three times and get the crude of salt-Dibazole.

5. Refinement

2 times of the crude of distilled water and the crude are added into the beaker, heat up to dissolve, the activated carbon is added and then filter out when the solution is hot, the filtrate is cooled and get the crystals, the crystals are ished by the distilled water three times, dry and test mp, calculate the yield.

6. Identification

(1) Infrared absorption spectroscopy; TLC counterpoint with standard substance.

(2) Nuclear magnetic resonance spectroscopy.

Notes:

1. *o*-phenylendiamine is dissolved by hydrochloric acid at 80-90℃, or the color of mono-salt *o*-phenylendimine turns deep and all the apparatuses are dried, the product is prepared and then the solvent is dried in the open air. The product is dried under the infrared lamp.

2. During the cyclization reaction, the odor is great, and the gas of jaws leads to the gullet, the speed of the rose temperature is ensured according to the speed of distilled water. At

the beginning, the temperature rises from 160℃ to 200℃, and maintains 200℃ for a long time, at last, half an hour, the temperature is 240℃, but not more than 240℃, or the yield is very low. After the temperature is below 150℃, the boiling water is added.

3. In the process of refinement, in order to remove unreacted phenyl acetic acid, crystals must be ished by a little water.

Questions

1. In the preparation of *o*-phenylendiamine, heat up a half of hydrochloric acid to boil, why is not the temperature too high?

2. What are the disadvantages when the temperature of the cyclization reaction is too high? Why?

3. Try to explain the mechanism of cyclization reation of benzimizole.

实验十七　亚胺－154 的合成

【目的要求】

掌握缩合、环合反应基本的操作和反应原理。

【实验原理】

亚胺－154 为抗肿瘤药物，对胃癌、肺癌等有一定的缓解作用，对肝癌、网状细胞肉瘤也有缓解作用，也用于银屑病（Psoriasis）的治疗。亚胺－154 化学名为 1,2-双(3,5-二氧哌-1 嗪)乙烷，化学结构式为：

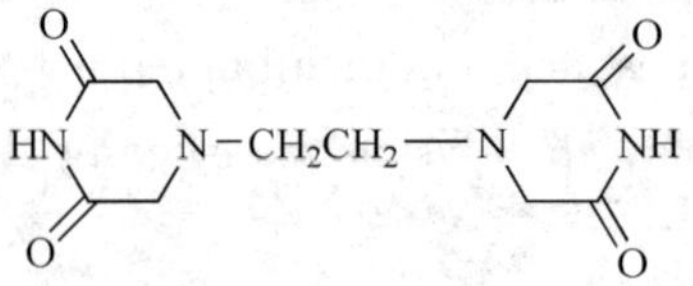

亚胺－154 为白色针状结晶。难溶于水及乙醇，碱中不稳定，mp. 290℃ ~292℃（分解）。

合成路线如下：

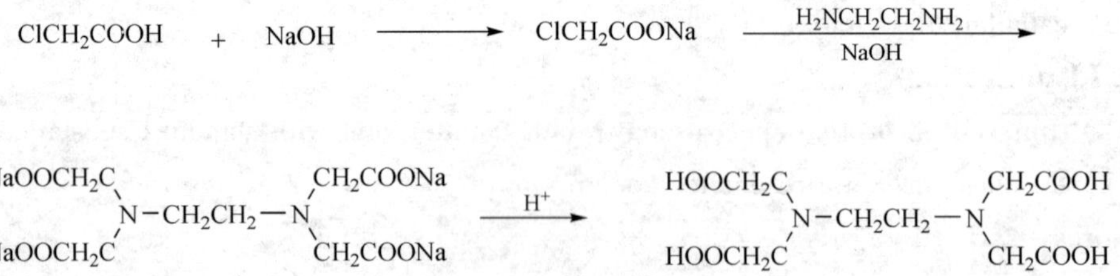

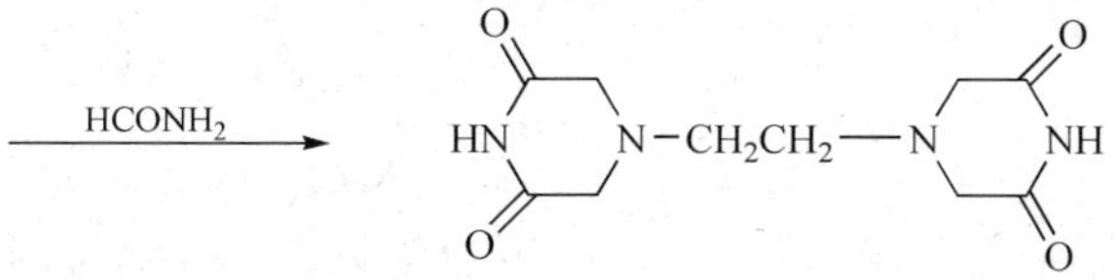

【实验方法】

（一）乙二胺四乙酸的制备

在装有温度计、搅拌器及滴液漏斗的 250 ml 三颈瓶中，投入氯乙酸 22. 5 g，加 45 ml水溶解。另将氢氧化钠 22 g 溶于 60 ml 水中，再加入乙二胺盐酸盐 6. 6 g，混匀后，置于滴液漏斗中，在搅拌下滴加到氯乙酸溶液中（约 1 ~2 min）。加料完毕后，温度上升至 102℃ ~106℃，pH 约为 9。将滴液漏斗换成冷凝器，搅拌保温 2 h。于前半小时内，分次测定反应液的 pH 值。当 pH 低于 9 时，补加少量 30% 氢氧化钠，使 pH 维持 9 左右。2 h 后，加入活性炭脱色，抽滤。滤液用盐酸酸化至 pH 1，放置，析出结晶，抽滤，结晶用水洗涤至氯离子呈阴性反应。干燥，得乙二胺四乙酸。熔点 210℃（分解）。

（二）乙二胺四乙酰亚胺的制备

将乙二胺四乙酸（eathylene diamine tetraacetic acid）14. 6 g，甲酰胺 26 g 置于装有搅拌器、温度计和直型冷凝器（除水用）的三颈瓶中。加热至 140℃左右，保温反应 90 min，再升温至 160℃ ±1℃，保温反应 4 h。反应过程中逸出的气体的 pH 由 3 逐渐上升，当升至 8 ~9 时，即为反应终点，趁热将反应液倒入冷水中，析出结晶，抽滤。结晶分别用水、乙醇洗涤，烘干，得乙二胺四乙酰亚胺白色结晶。mp. 295℃ ~300℃（分解）。

（三）结构确证

1. 红外吸收光谱法、标准物 TLC 对照法。

2. 核磁共振光谱法。

【思考题】

1. 在乙二胺和氯乙酸钠缩合反应中，为何 pH 控制在 9 左右。

2. 在乙二胺四乙酸与甲酰胺环合反应中，最初逸出的气体为何 pH 约为 3，而当结束时 pH 变为 8 ~9？

Experiment 17　Synthesis of Imine - 154

Purpose

To master the principle and basic operation of condensation and cyclization.

Mechanism

Imine - 154 is an antineoplastic agent, which can relieve the stomach and lung cancer, and it also relieves liver cancer and net cell sarcoma. It can be used in the treatment of psoriasis.

Its chemical name is 1,2-bis(3,5-dioxo-1-piperazinyl)ethane, and its structure is as follows:

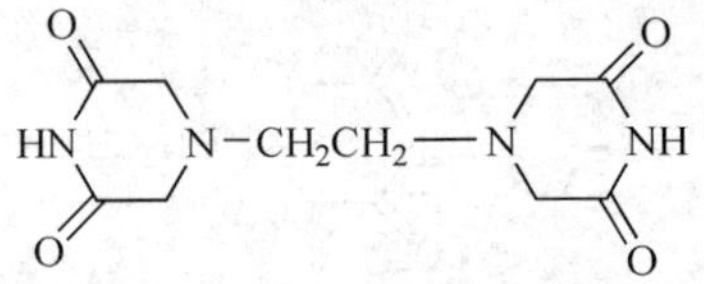

Imine－154 is a white needle crystal, insoluble in water and ethanol and unstable in base solution. mp. 290－292℃ (dec.).

The synthetic route is as follows:

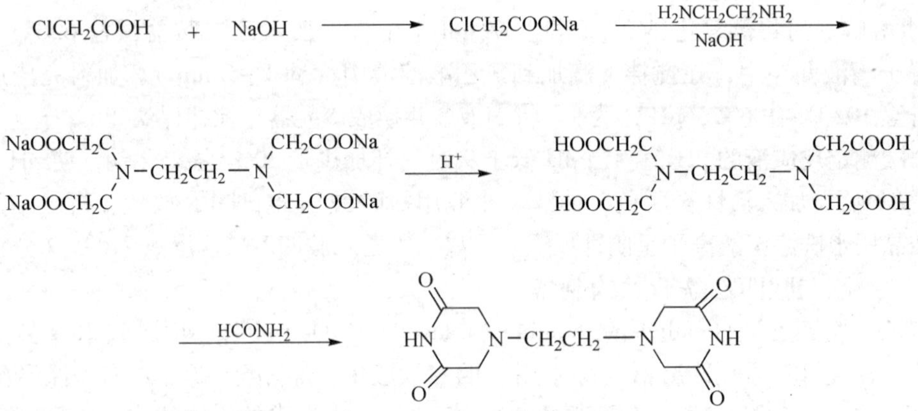

Experiment Procedure

1. The synthesis of Ethylene diamine tetraacetic acid (EDTA)

In a 250ml three-necked flask equipped with a stirrer, a thermometer and a dropping funnel 22.5 g of chloroacetic acid is added and dissolved in 45 ml of water. 22 g of sodium hydroxide is dissolved in 60 ml of water and 6.6 g of ethylenediamine hydrochloride is added. Then the mixture is transported in a dropping funnel and is dropped into the solution of the chloroacetic acid with stirring (about 1-2 min). Then the temperature is up to 102-106℃. and pH is 9. The dropping funnel is changed into a condenser, and the temperature is kept for 2 hours with stirring. Measured fractionally the pH of the solution within 0.5 hour. When the pH is below 9, a little of 30% sodium hydroxide is added in order to maintain the pH about 9. After 2 hours, some activated carbon is added to decolor the solution. Sucking filtrate, acidify the filtrate to pH 1 with hydrochloride and stand until the crystal is appeared. Filtrate, and ish with water until the detection of chloride ion is negative. Ethylene diamine tetraacetic acid is obtained after dried. mp: 210℃ (dec.).

2. The synthesis of Ethylenediamine Tetraacetylimide

In a three-necked flask equipped with a stirrer, a thermometer and a condenser, 14.6 g of ethylene diamine tetraacetic acid and 26 g of formamide are added. It is heated to 140℃ and is maintained at the temperature for 90 minutes. Then it is heated to 160℃ and is maintained at the temperature for 4 hours. The reaction is finished when the pH of the escaped gas rises from 3 to 8-9. Pour the hot reaction solution into cold water, and then precipitate the crystal. Suction filtrate, ish the product with water and ethanol, and dry it. The white crystal of ethylenediamine tetraacetylimide is obtained, mp 295-300℃ (dec.)

3. Identification

①Infrared absorption spectrometry, TLC confrontation method of the standard substance.

②Nuclear magnetic resonance spectroscopy.

Questions

1. Why should we control the pH about 9 in the condensation of ethylenediamine and sodium monochloroacetate?

2. Why is the pH of the escaped gas about 3 at first while the pH is 8-9 in the end during the cyclization of ethylene diamine tetraacetic acid and formamide?

实验十八　乙酰苯胺（Acetanilide）的合成

【目的要求】

1. 熟悉氨基酰化反应的原理及意义。
2. 掌握乙酰苯胺的制备方法。

【实验原理】

乙酰苯胺又称退热冰，是磺胺类药物的原料，可用作止痛剂、退热剂、防腐剂和染料中间体。

化学名：*N*-苯基乙酰胺

化学结构式：

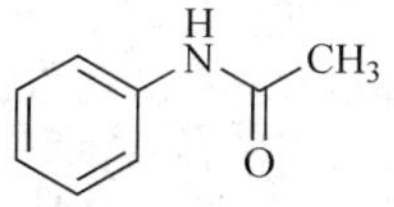

乙酰苯胺为白色有光泽片状结晶或白色结晶粉末，无臭或略有苯胺及乙酸气味，微溶于冷水，溶于热水、甲醇、乙醇、乙醚、三氯甲烷、丙酮等，不溶于石油醚。mp. 113℃～114℃。

合成路线如下：

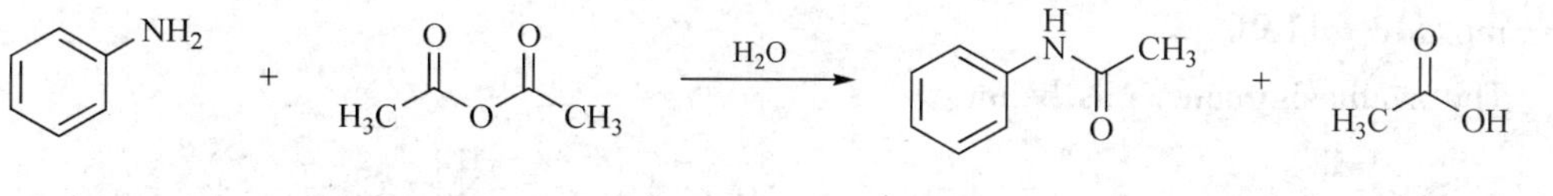

【实验方法】

（一）乙酰苯胺的制备

在250ml的三颈瓶上配置搅拌子、温度计、回流冷凝器及滴液漏斗，将10 ml苯胺及30 ml水加入反应瓶中，在搅拌下滴加14 ml乙酸酐，控制滴加速度以保证反应温度不超过40℃，随着乙酸酐的加入，析出白色固体，滴加完毕于室温继续搅拌30min，停止搅拌。室温下放置 10min，析晶完全，得到白色晶体，抽滤，以冷水洗涤滤饼 2 次，抽干，得乙酰苯胺粗品。计算收率。

（二）结构确证

1. 红外吸收光谱法、标准物 TLC 对照法。

2. 核磁共振光谱法。

[注释]

1. 此次用到的是两种液体反应原料，尤其是醋酐的刺激性较强，应建议在通风橱内量取，并且远离眼睛。

2. 滴加乙酸酐速度不能过快，防止剧烈放热，使苯胺氧化，使产品变黄或变红。若温度高（>35℃）可以在水浴锅中倒入冷水冷却。

【思考题】

1. 为何要控制乙酸酐的滴加速度？

2. 除了乙酸酐之外，还可以用哪些酰化试剂来制备乙酰苯胺？

Experiment 18 Synthesis of Acetanilide

Purpose

1. To study the principle and significance of amine acylation reaction

2. To master the preparation of acetanilide

Mechanism

Acetanilide is the raw material of sulfa drugs, can be used as an analgesic, antipyretic, antiseptic and dye intermediates, and so on.

Chemical name: *N*-phenylacetamide, and chemical structure is as follow:

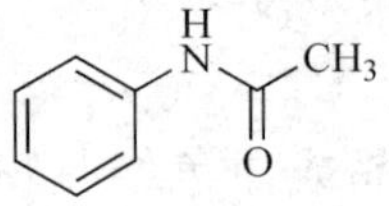

Acetanilide is a white luster flaky crystal or white crystalline powder, odorless and tasteless, or sightly aniline and acetic acid odour, slightly soluble in cold water, dissolve in hot water, methanol, ethanol, ethyl ether, chloroform, acetone and insoluble in petroleum ether. mp. 113 - 115℃.

The synthesis route is as below:

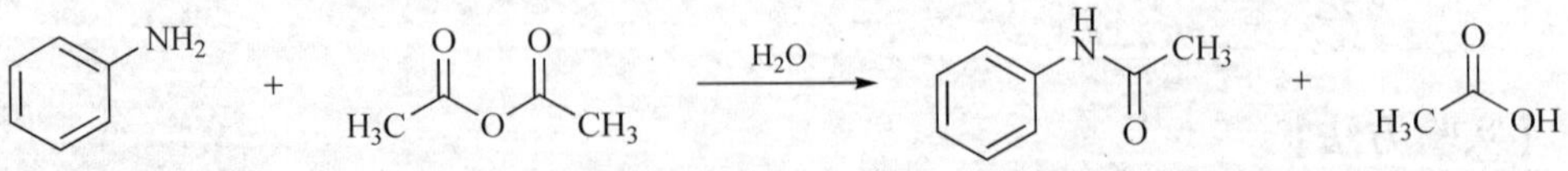

Experimental method

1. The preparation of acetanilide

In a 250ml three neck flask equipped with a stirrer, a thermometer, a reflux condenser and a dropping funnel, place 10 ml of aniline and 30 ml of water, drop 14 ml of acetic anhydride with stirring, control dropping speed to ensure that the reaction temperature is not more than 40℃. White solid precipitates with the addition of acetic anhydride. After dropping, continue stirring for 30 minutes at room temperature, stop stirring. At room temperature for 10 minutes, the complete crystallization gives white crystals, after crystallization precipitate completely, filtering, ishing twice with cold water, then pressed to dry, achieve crude acetanilide and the yield is calculated.

2. Structure Elucidation

（1） IR absorption spectroscopy, TLC standard material control law.

（2） NMR spectroscopy.

Notes:

（1） The two liquids are used as the reaction raw materials, especially strong irritant acetic anhydride, should be measured in a fume hood, and away from the eyes.

（2） Dropping speed of acetic anhydride can not be too fast to prevent violent exothermic, oxidation of aniline, the product yellow or red. If the temperature is high （ > 35℃）, the water bath can be poured into cold water to cool in the water bath.

Questions

1. Why do you want to control acetic anhydride dropping?

2. In addition to acetic anhydride, which acylating agent can be used to prepare acetanilide?

实验十九 乙酰苯胺（Acetanilide）的精制

【目的要求】

1. 学习重结晶的方法。

2. 学习熔点的测定方法。

【实验原理】

乙酰苯胺又称退热冰，是磺胺类药物的原料，可用作止痛剂、退热剂、防腐剂和染料中间体。利用乙酰苯胺粗品各组分在水中不同温度时的溶解度不同，从而实现乙酰苯胺的精制。

化学名：*N*-苯基乙酰胺

化学结构式：

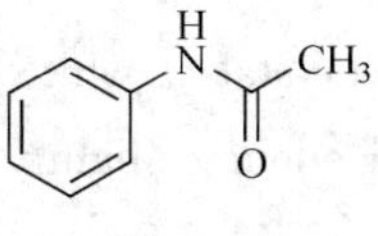

乙酰苯胺为白色有光泽片状结晶或白色结晶粉末，无臭或略有苯胺及乙酸气味，微溶于冷水，溶于热水、甲醇、乙醇、乙醚、三氯甲烷、丙酮等，不溶于石油醚。

mp. 113℃ ~114℃。

【实验方法】

（一）乙酰苯胺的重结晶

取乙酰苯胺粗品 2g 加入 90ml 水中，加入 1 粒沸石，加热至全溶后，稍冷，加入活性炭 0.2g，继续加热回流 10min。进行热过滤，将滤液转移至烧杯中，冷却，待析晶完全后抽滤，干燥，称重，计算收率。

（二）乙酰苯胺的熔点测定

测熔点，取少量乙酰苯胺精品在培养皿中研细，红外灯下充分干燥，将干燥好的固体粉末聚集成堆，装入熔点管，墩实，所装样品量大约为 2 ~3mm，固定熔点管的橡胶圈切勿进入硅油中，熔点管中的样品应处于温度计的水银球的中部，温度计应安装到 b 型管直管的中部，应在 b 型管的弯管部分加热，接近熔点时应控制温度每分钟上升 1℃ ~2℃，记录初熔温度和熔程。

（三）结构确证

1. 红外吸收光谱法、标准物 TLC 对照法。
2. 核磁共振光谱法。

【思考题】

1. 重结晶时加入沸石的目的是什么？
2. 重结晶时溶剂选择的标准是什么？
3. 简述熔点测定的一般操作方法。

Experiment 19 Refinement of Acetanilide

Purpose

1. To learn the recrystallization method.
2. To learn determination of the melting point.

Mechanism

Acetanilide is the raw material of sulfa drugs, can be used as an analgesic, antipyretic, antiseptic and dye intermediates, and so on.

Chemical name: *N*-phenylacetamide, and chemical structure is as follow:

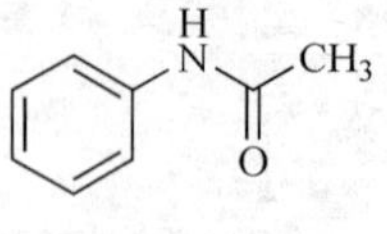

Acetanilide is a white luster flaky crystal or white crystalline powder, odorless and tasteless, or sightly aniline and acetic acid odour, slightly soluble in cold water, dissolve in hot water, methanol, ethanol, ethyl ether, chloroform, acetone and insoluble in petroleum ether, mp. 113-115℃.

Experiment method

1. The recrystallization of Acetanilide

Place 2 g of crude acetanilide to 90ml of water and add a grain of zeolite, heat to dissolve it. Cool the reaction mixture, and add 0. 2 g of activated carbon to bleach, reflux for 10 mins and filter. Filtrate will be transferred to the beaker, naturally cooling. After crystallization precipitate completely, filtering, pressure dryness, measure weight and yield.

2. The determination of the melting point

Place a small amount of pure acetanilide in petri dishes and porphyrize it, dry completely under infrared lamp. The dried powder gathers piles and is put into the melting point tubes, sample volume is about 2-3mm. The sample in melting point tubes should be in the middle of mercury bulb, a thermometer should be installed into the middle of straight tubes of b-type, heat elbow of b-type. When the tempreture is close to the melting point, control tempreture rise 1-2℃ per minute, record initial melting temperature and melting range.

3. Structure Elucidation

(1) IR absorption spectroscopy, TLC standard material control law.

(2) NMR spectroscopy.

Questions

1. What is the purpose of adding zeolite during recrystallization?
2. What is the solvent selection criteria during recrystallization?
3. Review the general operation ofmelting point determination.

实验二十 依达拉奉（Edaravone）的合成

【目的要求】

1. 掌握依达拉奉合成的基本原理。
2. 熟悉常压蒸馏、减压蒸馏和热抽滤等常用实验操作。

【实验原理】

依达拉奉（Edaravone）是一种脑保护剂（自由基清除剂）。临床用于治疗脑梗塞引起的神经病变。依达拉奉可清除自由基，抑制脂质过氧化，从而抑制脑细胞、血管内皮细胞、神经细胞的氧化损伤。

化学名：3-甲基-1-苯基-2-吡唑啉-5-酮

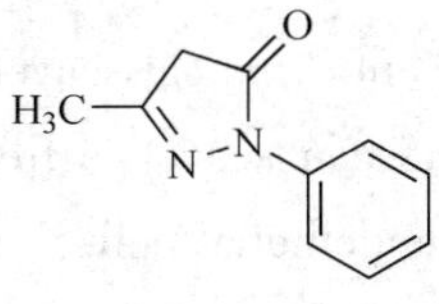

本品为白色或类白色结晶性粉末，无臭、无味。mp. 127. 5℃ ~128. 0℃，易溶于乙醇和乙酸，微溶于水。

合成路线如下：

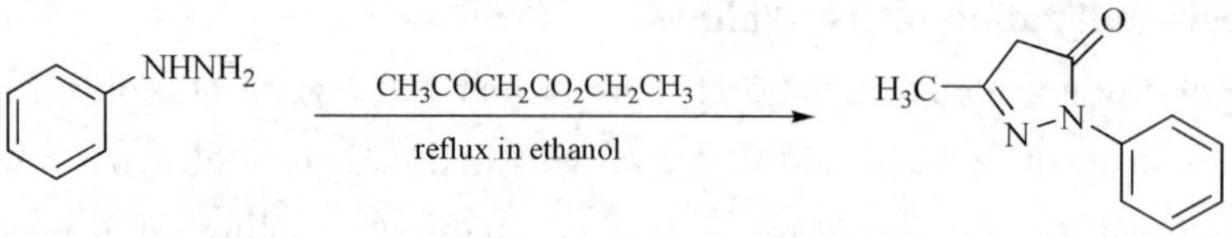

【实验方法】

（一）依达拉奉的制备

向装有球形冷凝管、滴液漏斗、磁力搅拌子和温度计的 250 ml 三颈瓶中，依次加入苯肼 14. 9 ml（150. 0 mmol）和无水乙醇 50 ml。室温下，向其中滴加乙酰乙酸乙酯 19. 1 ml（150. 0 mmol）。滴加完毕后，缓慢升温至回流，反应 4 h。改回流装置为蒸馏装置，缓慢蒸除乙醇至近干。稍冷，加乙酸乙酯 50 ml 并快速搅拌分散，逐渐析出固体。充分冷却，抽滤，以少量乙酸乙酯淋洗，转移固体，干燥，得淡黄色依达拉奉粗品。称重，计算收率。

（二）重结晶

取粗品 4. 0 g，置于装有球形冷凝管和磁力搅拌子的 100 ml 圆底瓶中，加入乙酸乙酯与乙醇（体积比 2∶1）的混和溶液 40 ml，升温至回流使粗品溶解。稍冷，加入活性炭 0. 5 g，继续回流脱色 15 min。趁热过滤，滤液冷却，析出颗粒状晶体，置于冰水浴中充分冷却。抽滤，干燥，得依达拉奉。称重，计算重结晶回收率。

【思考题】

1. 该缩合反应的机理？
2. 蒸馏乙醇过程为什么要缓慢，其目的是什么？
3. 本反应可能发生哪些副反应、产生的副产物？
4. 依达拉奉精制时选择溶媒的依据？如何提高重结晶的回收率？

Experiment 20　Synthesis of Edaravone

Purpose

1. To learn the reaction mechanism of the synthesis of Edaravone.

2. To master the use of atmospheric and vacuum distillation，filtration and other commonly used experimental operation.

Mechanism

Edaravone is a neuroprotective agent（radical scavenger）for the treatment of cerebral infarction induced neuropathy. Edaravone can scavenge free radicals and inhibit lipid peroxidation，thereby inhibiting brain cells，endothelial cells，oxidative damage to nerve cells.

Chemical name：3-methyl-1-phenyl-2-pyrazolin-5-one，and chemical structure is as follow：

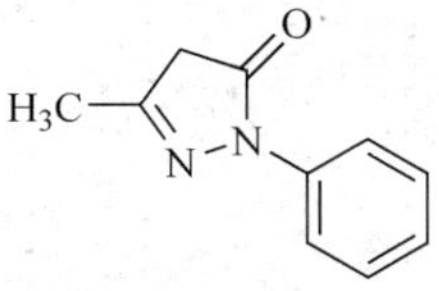

Edaravone regards as a white or almost white crystalline powder, odorless, tasteless. mp. 127. 5-128. 0℃. It is soluble in ethanol and acetic acid, slightly soluble in water.

The synthetic route is as follow:

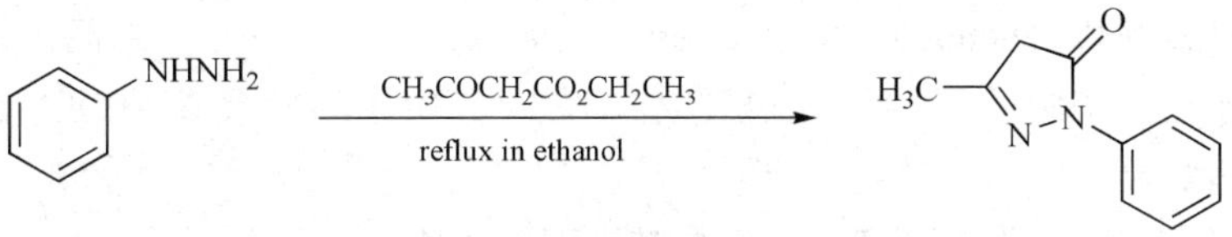

Experiment method

1. The preparation of Edaravone

To a 250 ml three-neck flask with a spherical condenser, a dropping funnel, a thermometer and a magnetic stirrer were added 14. 9 ml (150. 0 mmol) of phenylhydrazine and 50 ml of ethanol. Then 19. 1 ml (150. 0 mmol) of ethyl acetoacetate ester was slowly added at room temperature. After the addition, the reaction mixture was slowly heated to reflux, and reacted under refluxing for 4 h. The ethanol was slowly distilled off *via* atmospheric distillation. After immediate addition of 50 ml of ethyl acetate, it was quickly stirred, and white crystalline solid gradually appeared. The solid was filtered, washed with a little ethyl acetate, and dried to afford the crude. The dried crude was weighed for the yield calculation.

2. Recrystallization

The crude 4. 0 g was added into a 100 ml round bottom flask with a spherical condenser and a magnetic stirrer, then 40 ml of ethyl acetate/ethanol ($V/V = 2:1$) was added. The mixture was heated to reflux to dissolve the solid. After cooled for a while, 0. 5 g of activated carbon was added to the mixture. It was reheated for refluxing for about 15 min, then filtered.

The mother liquid was cooled to give granular crystalline precipitate. It was treated with an ice bath for complete precipitation. The crystal was collected *via* vacuum filtration, dried to give the final product. It was weighed to calculate the yield of this procedure.

Questions

1. The mechanism of the condensation reaction.

2. Why should the ethanol be slowly distilled off after the reaction, and its purpose?

3. To state the possible side reactions, and the corresponding by-products.

4. The main consideration of the solvent selection for the recrystallization? How to improve the recovery yield of the process?

实验二十一　盐酸苯海索（Benzhexol Hydrochloride）的合成

【目的要求】

1. 了解 Grignard 反应、Mannich 反应的机理以及在药物合成中的应用。
2. 掌握 Grignard 试剂的制备方法与无水操作步骤。

【实验原理】

盐酸苯海索（Benzhenol Hydrochloride）又名安坦（Antane）。本品能阻断中枢神经系统和周围神经系统中的毒碱样胆碱受体。临床上用于治疗震颤麻痹综合症，也用于斜颈、颜面痉挛等。

化学名：1-环已基-1-苯基-3-(1-哌啶基)-丙醇盐酸盐

化学结构式：

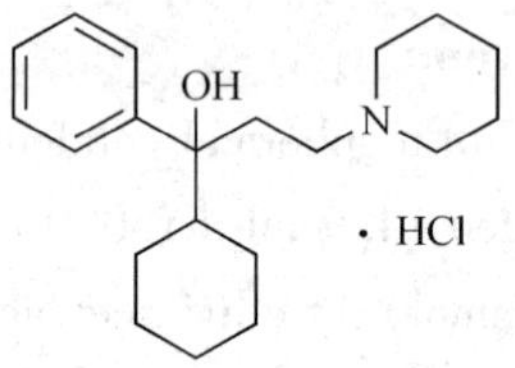

该品为白色晶体，熔点：250℃ ~256℃，在甲醇，乙醇和三氯甲烷中溶解，在水中微溶。

合成路线如下：

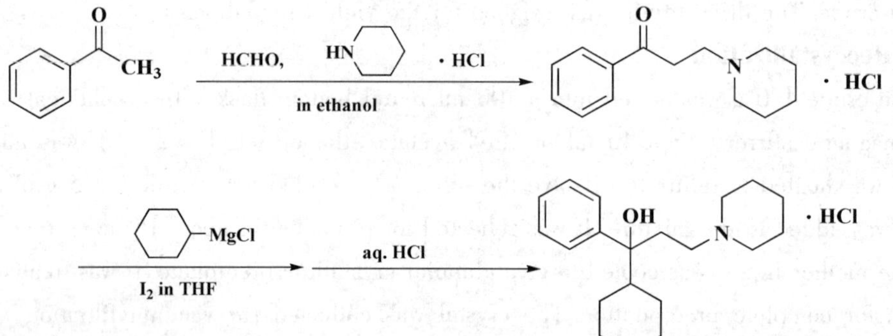

【实验方法】

（一）β-哌啶基苯丙酮盐酸盐的制备

在装有磁力搅拌子、温度计和球形冷凝器的 250 ml 三颈瓶中，依次加入苯乙酮 18.02 g（150.0 mmol）、95%乙醇 40 ml、哌啶盐酸盐 18.24 g（150.0 mmol）、多聚甲醛 7.65 g（85.0 mmol）和浓盐酸 0.5 ml，搅拌回流 3 h。以冷水冷却反应液，逐渐析出固体。抽滤，乙醇洗涤至中性，干燥，得白色鳞片状结晶，mp. 190℃ ~194℃。称重，计算收率。

（二）盐酸苯海索粗品的制备

向装有电磁搅拌、温度计、滴液漏斗和上方附有塑料气球的球型冷凝器的 250 ml 三颈瓶中，依次投入镁屑 4. 32 g（180. 0 mmol）、四氢呋喃 80 ml、少量碘。加入约总量 1/4 量的氯代环己烷与四氢呋喃的溶液后，缓慢升温至 50℃左右以引发该反应，当碘的颜色褪去且反应液保持微沸状态时，表示反应已经开始。随后慢慢滴入余下的氯代环己烷的四氢呋喃，累计加入氯代环己烷 14. 23 g（120. 0 mmol）及四氢呋喃 20 ml，滴加速度以保持微沸状态为准。加毕，继续回流 30 min，至反应不再进行。然后用冷水冷却，搅拌下分次加入哌啶基苯丙酮盐酸盐 25. 38 g（100. 0 mmol），约 20 min 内加完，再搅拌回流 2 h。将反应液冷却至室温，搅拌下将其缓慢倾倒至冷的 3. 0 mol/L 稀盐酸溶液约 80 ml 中，搅拌片刻，继续冰水浴冷却使固体充分析出。抽滤，以水洗至 pH =5。干燥，得盐酸苯海索粗品。称重，计算收率。

（三）粗品的重结晶

粗品以 1. 0 ~1. 5 倍量（*V/W*）乙醇重结晶。加热溶解，活性炭脱色，趁热过滤。滤液以冰水浴冷却，充分析晶。抽滤，干燥，得盐酸苯海索纯品，mp. 250℃ ~256℃。称重，计算重结晶回收率。

（四）结构确证

1. 红外吸收光谱法、标准物 TLC 对照法。
2. 核磁共振光谱法。

[注释]

1. 反应中有氯化氢气体逸出，需以塑料气球捕捉酸性气体。
2. 格式试剂制备和格氏反应中所用的仪器及试剂必须充分干燥。
3. 镁屑的外层常被灰色氧化镁覆盖，应先以稀盐酸快速处理、蒸馏水洗、乙醇洗迅速放入烘箱中进行减压干燥。
4. Grignard 反应后，应缓慢倾倒至稀酸中，以免后处理过于激烈。

【思考题】

1. 写出上述 Mannich 反应的反应机理。
2. 制备 Grignard 试剂时，加入少量碘的作用是什么？
3. 本实验的 Mannich 反应为何在酸性下进行？

Experiment 21 Synthesis of Benzhexol Hydrochloride

Purpose

1. Familiar with the mechanism of Grignard reaction and Mannich reaction and their application in the pharmaceutical synthesis.

2. To master the preparation method of Grignard agent and the operation under water-free condition.

Mechanism

Benzhenol Hydrochloride, also known as Antane, can inhibit the muscarine-type cholinergic receptors in the central and peripheral nervous system with clinical treatment for the Parkinsonism syndrome, torticollis and facial spasm, etc.

Its chemical name is 1-cyclohexyl-1-phenyl-3-(1-piperidinyl) propan-1-ol hydrochloride, and its chemical structure is as follow:

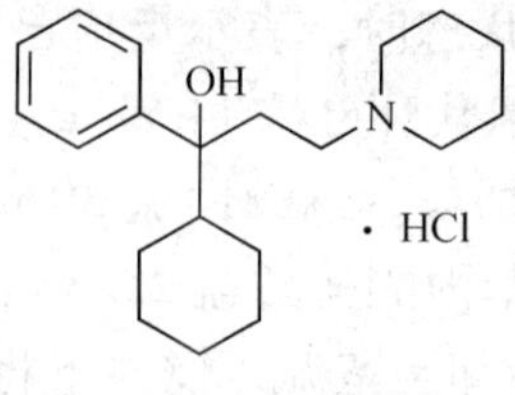

Benzhenol Hydrochloride is a white crystal with melting point 250-256℃, and soluble in the methanol, enthanol and chloroform, while slightly soluble in the water.

The synthetic route is as follow:

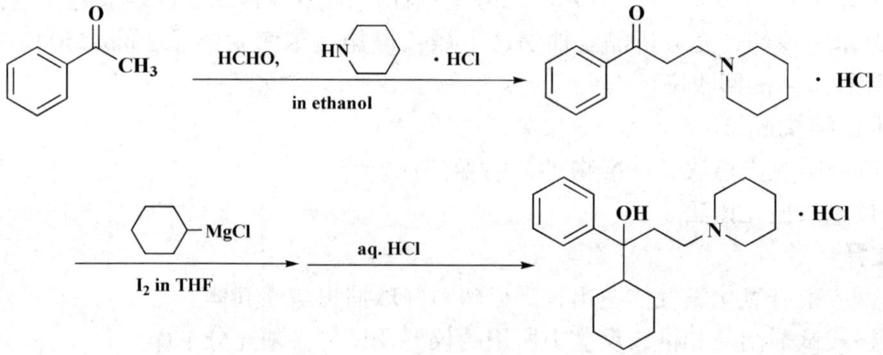

Experiment method

1. The preparation of 1-phenyl-3-(1-piperidinyl) propan-1-one

To a 250ml three-necked flask equipped with a magnetic stirrer, a thermometer and a reflux condenser were added 18.02 g (150.0 mmol) of acetophenone, 40 ml of 95% ethanol, 18.24 g (150.0 mmol) of piperidine hydrochloride, 7.65 g (85.0 mmol) of paraformaldehyde and 0.5 ml of concentrated hydrochloric acid in order. It was stirred under refluxing for 3 h. After cooled with cool water, the solid intermediate was precipitated from the system. The solid was collected via filtration, washed with ethanol till neutral to obtain flake white crystalline product, mp. 190-194℃. It was weighed to calculate the yield.

2. Preparation of crude Benzhenol Hydrochloride

To a 250 ml three-necked flask equipped with a magnetic stirrer, a thermometer, a dropping funnel and a reflux condenser with a balloon on the top were added successively 4.32 g of magnesium spalls (180.0 mmol), 80 ml of tetrahydrofuran, and a small amount of iodine. About one-fourth of the chlorocyclohexane was introduced through the funnel, then the mixture was heated to about 50℃ till the color of the iodine faded and the reaction liquid kept micro-boiling indicating the initiation of the Grignard reaction. The remaining mixture of chlorocyclohexane in THF was added into the system while keeping the reaction under refluxing. The total amount of chlorocyclohexane 21. 35 g(180. 0 mmol) in 20 ml of tetrahydrofuran was used for the preparation. After the addition, it was refluxed for about 30 mins until the magnesium spalls disappeared. It was cooled with water, 25. 38 g (100. 0 mmol) of 1-phenyl-3-(1-piperidinyl) propan-1-one prepared above was added in portions in 20 mins. The mixture was refluxed for another 2 h, re-cooled to room temperature, and at last poured into 80 ml of 3. 0 mol/L hydrochloric acid. It was stirred for a while, and cooled with ice-water bath for completing precipitation. The solid was collected via filtration, washed with water till pH = 5. The dried crude benzhenol hydrochloride was weighed to calculate the yield.

3. Purification of the crude

The crude was recrystallized in 1. 0-1. 5 ratio of ethanol (*V/W*). It was heated until dissolved, and treated with activated carbon. Then it was filtrated, and the filtrate was cooled with ice-water. The solid was collected and dried to afford the final product. Its melting point was 250-256℃. It was weighed to calculate the recovery yield of the process.

4. Identification

① Infrared absorption spectrometry, standard comparison method of TLC chromatography.

② Nuclear magnetic resonance spectroscopy.

Notes:

(1) A plastic balloon was used to trap the produced hydrogen chloride.

(2) The glassware and the reagents should be fully dried in the preparation of Grignard reagent and the successive Grignard reaction.

(3) It was recommended that the magnesium spalls should be quickly pretreated with diluted hydrochloric acid to remove gray magnesium oxide on the surface. Then it was filtered, washed with water and then with ethanol, and quickly dried under vacuum.

(4) After the Grignard reaction, it was cautiously poured into the diluted hydrochloric acid in case of vigorous reaction.

Questions

1. Give the mechanism of the above Mannich reaction.
2. Explain the effect of the small amount of iodine in the preparation for Grignard agent.
3. Why should the Mannich reaction proceed under acidic condition?

实验二十二　奥沙普秦（Oxaprozin）的合成

【实验目的】

1. 掌握奥沙普秦的反应机理。
2. 学习合成奥沙普秦的实验操作。

【实验原理】

奥沙普秦适用于风湿性关节炎、类风湿性关节炎、强直性脊柱炎、肩关节周围炎、颈肩腕症喉群、痛风发作以及外伤和手术后消炎、镇痛。

化学名：4,5-二苯基噁唑-2-丙酸。

化学结构式：

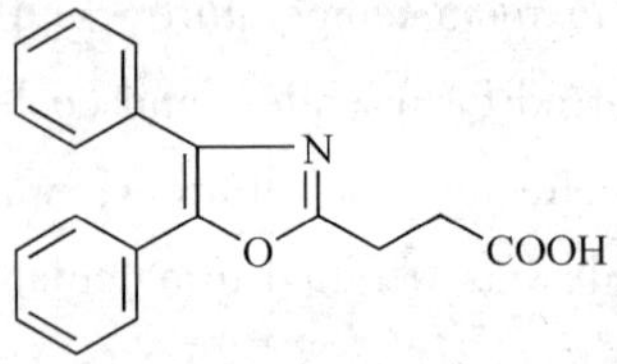

本品用甲醇重结晶得白色晶体，无臭、味微苦。mp. 160. 5℃ ~161. 5℃，易溶于二甲基甲酰胺和二氧六环，略溶于乙醇。

合成路线如下：

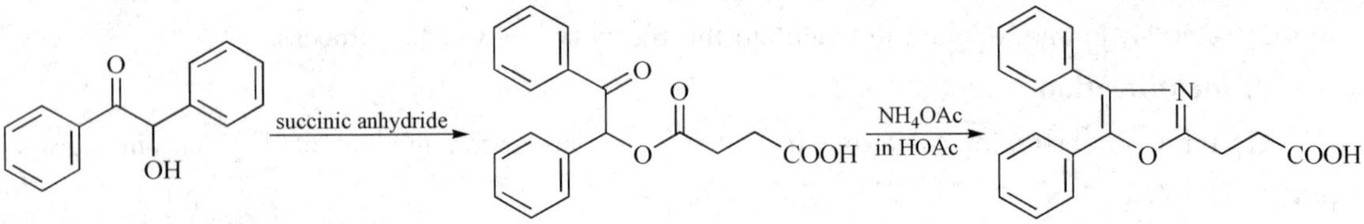

【实验方法】

（一）安息香琥珀酸酯的制备

在装有搅拌子、温度计和附有干燥管的球形冷凝器的 100 ml 三颈瓶中，依次加入丁二酸酐 4. 00 g（40. 0 mmol），安息香 8. 40 g（40. 0 mmol）。加毕，搅拌下，缓慢将内温升至 120℃，并保温反应 4 h，冷却至室温，直接投下一步。

（二）奥沙普秦的制备

向上一步装有搅拌子、温度计和附有干燥管的球形冷凝器的 100 ml 三颈瓶中，加入冰乙酸 40. 0 ml 和乙酸铵 10. 0 g（130. 0 mmol）。加热至 120℃，搅拌反应 4 h。冷却至室温，将反应液倾倒入含有 40 ml 水的 100 ml 烧杯中，析出固体。抽滤，以少量水淋洗滤饼，干燥，计算收率。

（三）精制

粗品以 2. 0 ~2. 5 倍量（*V/W*）甲醇重结晶。加热溶解，活性炭脱色 0. 5 h，趁热抽滤。室温搅拌析晶，待析出固体后，以冰水浴冷却，充分析晶。抽滤，干燥。称重，计算重结晶回收率。

（四）结构确证

1. 红外吸收光谱法、标准物 TLC 对照法。
2. 核磁共振光谱法。

【思考题】

1. 写出环合反应制备奥沙普秦的反应机理。
2. 探讨以上精制方法的原理，并简述活性炭脱色的目的所在。

Experiment 22　Synthesis of Oxaprozin

Purpose

1. To master the principle and the basic operation for the synthesis of oxaprozin.

2. To master the experimental procedure for the synthesis of oxaprozin.

Mechanism

Oxaprozin can be used for the treatments of rheumatoid arthritis, rheumatoid arthritis, ankylosing spondylitis, inflammation around the shoulder, neck and wrist disorders throat group, gout attacks. It can also be used for post-traumatic and surgical anti-inflammatory and analgesic.

Chemical name: 3-(4,5-diphenyloxazol-2-yl) propanoic acid, and the chemical structure is as follow:

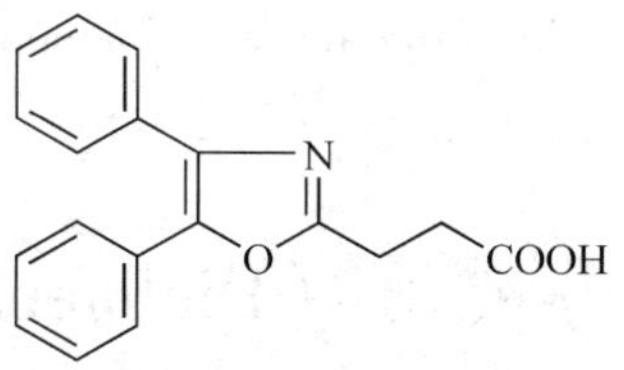

Oxaprozin is a needle-like crystal, odorless, mildly bitter flavor. mp. 160.5-161.5℃. It is soluble in DMF and dioxane, slightly soluble in ethanol.

The synthetic route is as follows:

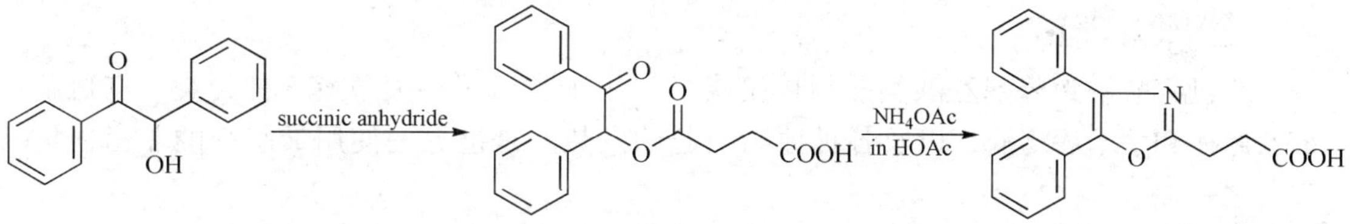

Experiment method

1. The preparation of benzoin hemisuccinate

To a dry 100 ml three-necked flask equipped with a stirrer bar, a thermometer and a reflux condenser with a calcium chloride drier on the top, was added successively 4.00 g (40.0 mmol) of succinic anhydride, 8.40 g (40.0 mmol) of benzoin. After the addition, the mixture was heated with stirring at 120℃ for 4 h. It was cooled for a while.

2. The preparation of oxaprozin

To the above 100 ml three-necked flask equipped with a stirrer bar, a thermometer and a reflux condenser with a calcium chloride drier on the top, was added 40.0 ml of glacial acetic acid and 10.0 g(130 mmol) of ammonium acetate. The mixture was then reheated at 120℃ for another 4 h. The reaction mixture was cooled to room temperature. It was poured into a 100 ml beaker containing 40 ml of water. The formed solid was filtered, washed with a little water and dried. The crude was weighed to calculate the yield.

3. The refinement

The crude was recrystallized in 2. 0-2. 5 ratio of methanol(*V/W*). It was heated until dissolved, and treated with activated carbon. Then it was filtrated, and the filtrate was cooled with ice-water. The solid was collected and dried to afford the final product. It was weighed to calculate the recovery yield of the process.

4. Identification

(1) Infrared absorption spectrometry, TLC confrontation method of the standard substance.

(2) Nuclear magnetic resonance spectroscopy.

Questions

1. Write the possible mechanism of the cyclization for the preparation of oxaprozin?

2. Try to understand the principle of the above refinement, and to know the purpose of the addition of activated carbon.

实验二十三　双氯芬酸钠（Diclofenac Sodium）的合成

【目的要求】

1. 通过双氯芬酸钠的制备，了解酰化试剂的选择依据及操作中的注意事项。

2. 掌握 Friedel－Crafts 反应的反应原理。

【实验原理】

双氯芬酸钠为芳基乙酸类非甾体抗炎药，用于类风湿性关节炎、神经炎、红斑狼疮及癌症和手术后疼痛，以及各种原因引起的发热。是世界上使用最广泛的非甾体抗炎药之一。

化学名：2-(2,6-二氯苯基)氨基苯乙酸钠

化学结构式：

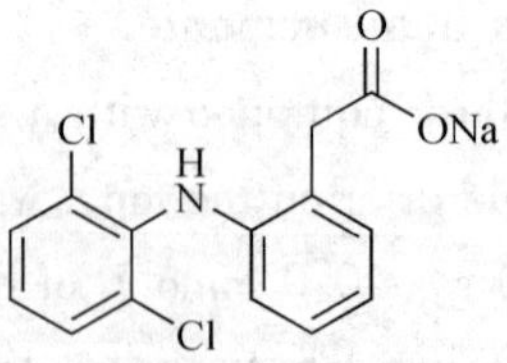

双氯芬酸钠为白色或类白色结晶性粉末，无臭，略溶于水，易溶于乙醇。mp. 283℃～285℃。

合成路线如下：

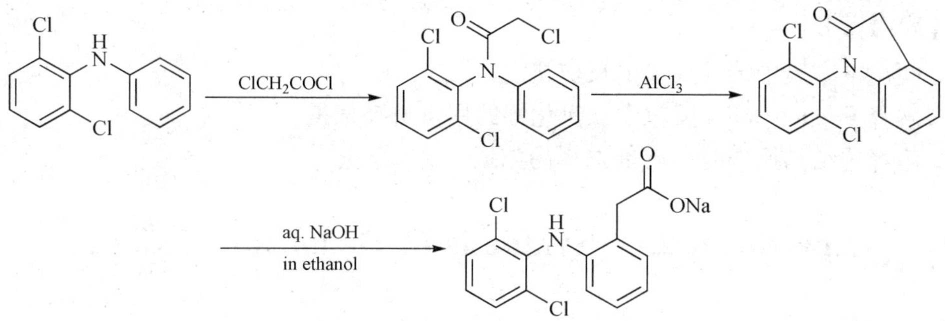

【实验方法】

（一）*N*-苯基-*N*-(2,6-二氯苯基)氯乙酰胺的制备

向装有电磁搅拌、温度计、附有塑料气球的球形冷凝管的100 ml三颈瓶中，依次加入2,6-二氯二苯胺11.91 g（0.05 mol）和氯乙酰氯4.75 ml（0.06 mol）。搅拌下，缓慢将内容物加热升温至140 C，并保温反应2 h，过程中产生的酸性气体以气球收集。停止加热，待内容物降温至40℃～50℃之后，再向其中缓慢补加95 %乙醇15 ml，分解过量的氯乙酰氯、溶解有色杂质。冷却至室温，再冰水浴冷却充分析晶。抽滤，少量乙醇洗，干燥，得粗品，mp. 143℃～144℃，计算收率。

（二）1-(2,6-二氯苯基)二氢吲哚-2-酮的制备

向装有电磁搅拌、温度计、附有塑料气球的球形冷凝管的100 ml三颈瓶中，加入上步所制粗品12.59 g（0.04 mol）、无水三氯化铝10.67 g（0.08 mol），加热升温，待反应物熔融后开始搅拌，继续升温至150℃，并保温反应3 h。冷却至室温后，将反应混和物缓慢倒入装有150 ml冰水的烧杯中进行水解，边倒边搅拌，逐渐析出固体。冰水浴下充分冷却，抽滤，少量水（5 ml×2）淋洗，干燥，得粗品，mp. 124℃～125℃，计算收率。

（三）双氯芬酸钠的制备

向装有电磁搅拌、温度计和球形冷凝管的100 ml三颈瓶中，加入上步所制粗品5.56 g（0.02 mol）、2.5 mol/L氢氧化钠溶液20 ml（0.05 mol）、乙醇溶液20 ml。将反应混和物搅拌回流3 h，冷却析晶，抽滤、少量水淋洗，得粗品，mp. 283℃～285℃，计算收率。

（四）精制

向装有电磁搅拌和球形冷凝管的100 ml圆底瓶中，加入双氯芬酸钠粗品4.00 g和0.2 mol/L氢氧化钠溶液30 ml，搅拌升温至85℃直至固体溶解。加入活性炭0.50 g，继续保温脱色30 min，趁热过滤。滤液冷却析晶，过滤，少量水淋洗，干燥，得产品，计算收率。

（五）结构确证

1. 红外吸收光谱法、标准物TLC对照法。
2. 核磁共振光谱法。

【思考题】

1. 写出本实验中涉及反应的反应机理。
2. 解释 Friedel-Crafts 反应中三氯化铝的用量选择依据。
3. 解释重结晶操作时，溶剂选择的依据。

Experiment 23　Synthesis of Diclofenac Sodium

Purpose

1. To comprehend the principle of the selection of acylating reagent in the synthesis of Diclofenac Sodium, to understand the cautions in the operating process.

2. To master the mechanism of the Friedel-Crafts reaction.

Mechanism

Diclofenac is an aryl acetic acid non-steroidal anti-inflammatory drug, which is used for the treatment of rheumatoid arthritis, neuritis and lupus, and for the relief of cancer pain or surgery pain. It is one of the world's most widely used non-steroidal anti-inflammatory drugs.

Chemical name is sodium 2-[(2,6-dichlorophenyl)amino]benzeneacetic acid, and its chemical structure is as follow:

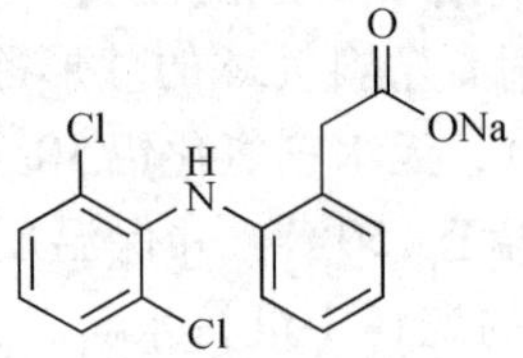

Sodium diclofenac is a white or almost white crystalline powder with melting point of 283-285℃. It is odorless solid which is slightly soluble in water, soluble in ethanol.

Thesynthetic route is as below:

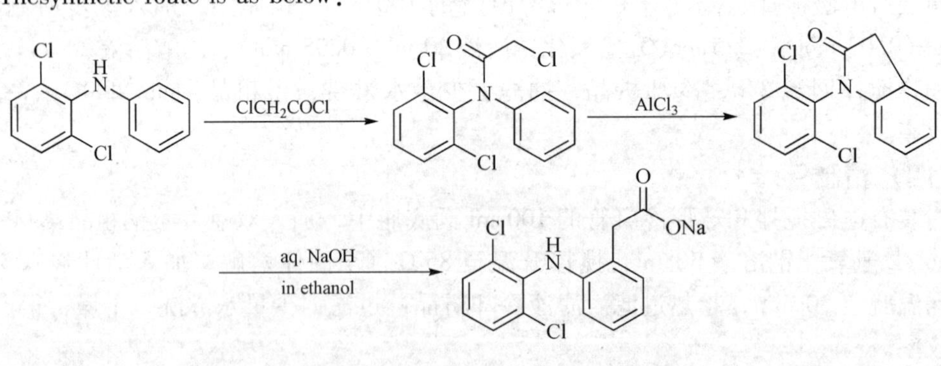

Experiment method

1. Preparation of *N*-(2,6-Dichlorophenyl)-*N*-phenylchloroacetamide

To a 100 ml dried three-necked flask equipped with an agitator, a thermometer and a reflux condenser with a plastic balloon on the top, was added 11.91 g (50 mmol) of 2,6-dichlorodiphenylamine and 4. 8 ml (60 mmol) of chloroacetyl chloride. The mixture was heated in an oil bath at 140℃ for 2 h, and the acid gas was trapped with the balloon. Then it was cooled until 40-50℃, and 15 ml of 95% ethanol was added to decompose the excessive chloroacetyl chloride and to dissolve the color impurities. It was first cooled to room temperature and then with an ice-water bath to completely precipitate the solid. After filtration, the solid was washed with a little ethanol and dried. The crude, mp. 143-144℃, is weighed to calculate the yield.

2. Preparation of 1-(2,6-dichlorophenyl)-2-indolinone

To a 100 ml dried three-necked flask equipped with a stirrer, a thermometer and a reflux condenser with a plastic balloon on the top, was added the above amide 12. 60 g (40 mmol) and anhydrous aluminum chloride 10. 67 g(80 mmol). After the addition, the mixture was heated in an oil bath. It could be stirred until the starting material melted, and the mixture was continually heated up to 150℃ and stirred at the temperature for 3 h. After it was cooled to room temperature, the reaction mixture was poured into 150 ml of ice water while stirring, and the solid precipitated from the system. After sufficienthy cooled with an ice-water bath, the solid was collected by filtration, washed with water, and dried. The crude, mp. 124-125℃, was weighed to calculate the yield.

3. Preparation of Diclofenac Sodium

To a 100 ml dried three-necked flask equipped with a stirrer, a thermometer and a reflux condenser, was added 5. 56 g(20 mmol) of the above lactam, 20 ml(50 mmol) of 2. 5 mol/L sodium hydroxide solution and 20 ml of ethanol. The mixture was refluxed for 3 h, it was cooled for crystallization. The solid was filtered, washed with a little water. The dried crude, mp. 283-285℃, is weighed to calculate the yield of this hydrolysis.

4. Refinement

To a 100 ml dried flask equipped with a stirrer, and a reflux condenser, was added the crude 3. 60 g(15 mmol), and 30 ml(6 mmol) of 0. 20 mol/L sodium hydroxide solution. The mixture was heated with an oil bath to about 85℃ until the crude was dissolved. After the addition of 0. 50 g of activated carbon, the mixture was stirred for another 30 mins. It was filtered, cooled for sufficient crystallization. The solid was collected by filtration, washed with a small amount of water. The dried product was weighed to calculate the yield of this recrystallization.

5. Identification

(1) Infrared absorption spectrometry, TLC confrontation method of the standard substance.

(2) Nuclear magnetic resonance spectroscopy.

Questions

1. Please write the mechanism of the above related reactions.

2. Please give a reasonable explanation of the amount of aluminum chloride used in this

experiment.

3. Please comment on the selection of solvents for this recrystallization.

实验二十四　诺氟沙星（Norfloxacin）的合成

【目的要求】

1. 通过对诺氟沙星合成，对新药研制过程有一基本认识。

2. 通过对诺氟沙星合成路线的比较，掌握选择实际生产工艺的几个基本要求。

3. 通过实际操作，对涉及到的各类反应特点、机制、操作要求、反应终点的控制等，进一步巩固有机化学试验的基本操作，领会掌握理论知识。

4. 掌握各部中间体的质量控制方法。

【实验原理】

诺氟沙星的化学名为1-乙基-6-氟-1,4-二氢-4-氧-7-(1-哌嗪基)-3-喹啉羧酸，1-ethyl-6-fluoro-1,4-dihydro-4-oxo-7-(1-piperazinyl)-3-quino-linecarboxylic acid，化学结构式为：

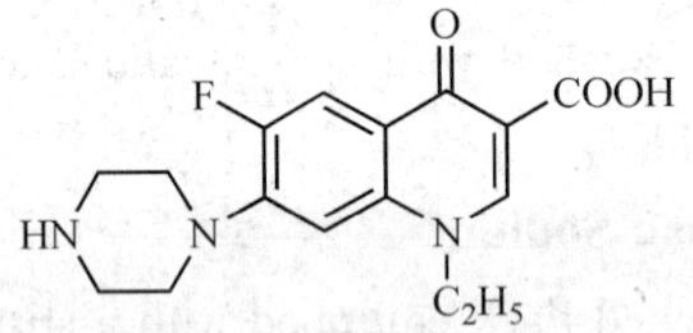

诺氟沙星为微黄色针状晶体或结晶性粉末，mp. 216℃ ~220℃，易溶于酸及碱，为溶于水。

诺氟沙星的制备方法很多，按不同原料及路线划分可有十几种。我国工业生产以路线一为主。近几年来，许多新工艺在诺氟沙星生产中获得应用，其中以路线二，即硼螯合物法收率高，操作简便，单耗低，且质量较好。

合成路线如下：

路线一：

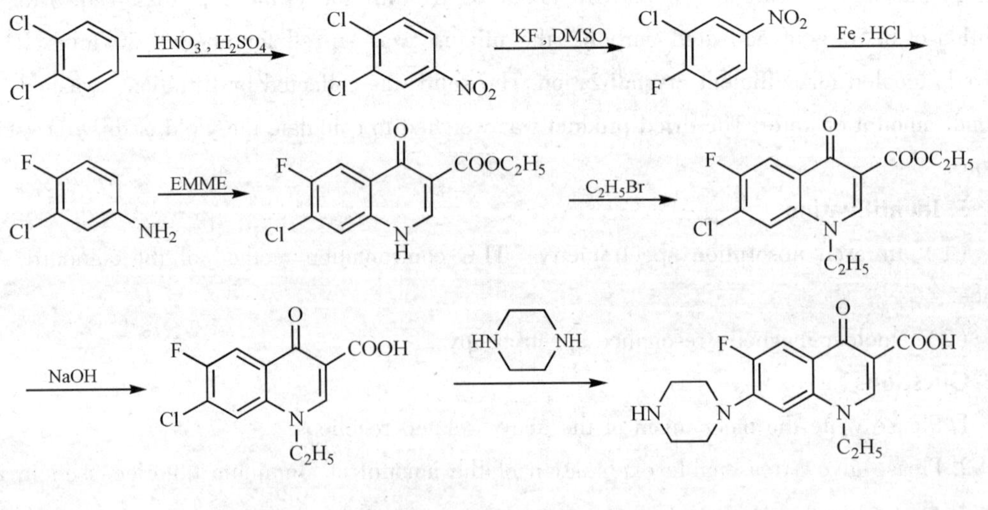

路线二：

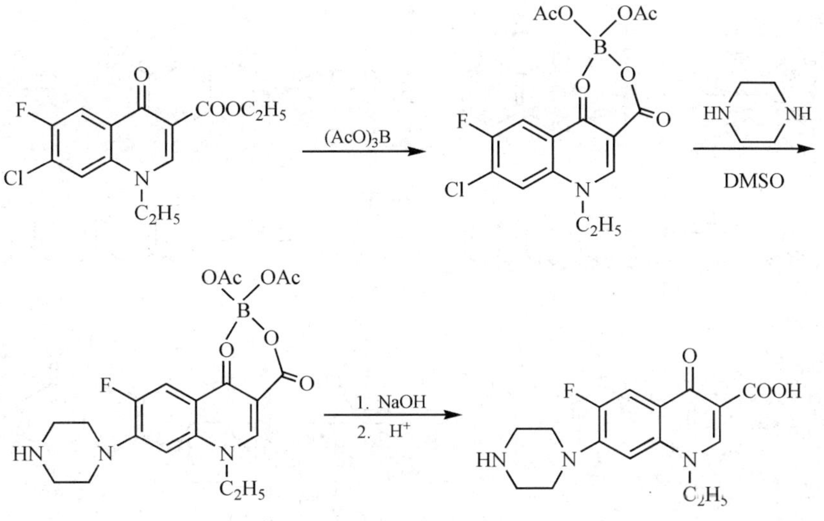

Experiment 24　Synthesis of Norfloxacin

Purpose

1. To understand generally the new medicine research through the synthesis of Norfloxacin.

2. To master the basic requests for choosing actual production craft through comparison of the synthesis route.

3. Through the actual operation, referring to each kind of reacting characteristic, the mechanism, the operation request, the control of the end of point and so on, further consolidate the basic operation and elementary operation as well as grasp the theory.

4. To grasp the quality controlling method of each intermediate.

Mechanism

Norfloxacin is also named 1-ethyl-6-fluoro-14-dihydro-4-oxo-7-(1-piperazinyl)-3-quinolinecarboxylic acid. Its structure as follows:

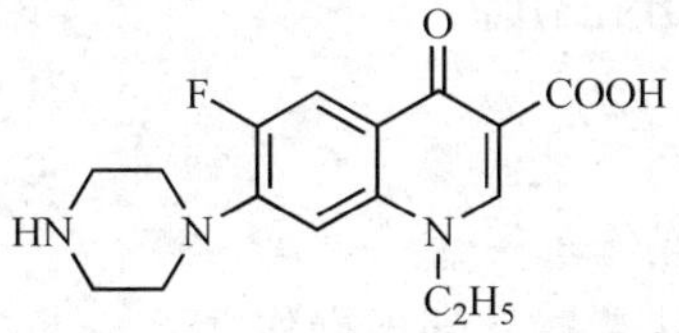

Norfloxacin is light yellow needles or minute crystals, soluble in acid and base.

There are many ways to prepare Norfloxacin, may have several kinds according to raw material and the route. Our country industrial production primarily uses route 1. In the last few years, many new techniques had been applied to prepare norfloxacin, such as route 2, boron chelated complex has high rate, simple operation, low loss and good quality.

The synthetic route is as follows：

Route 1：

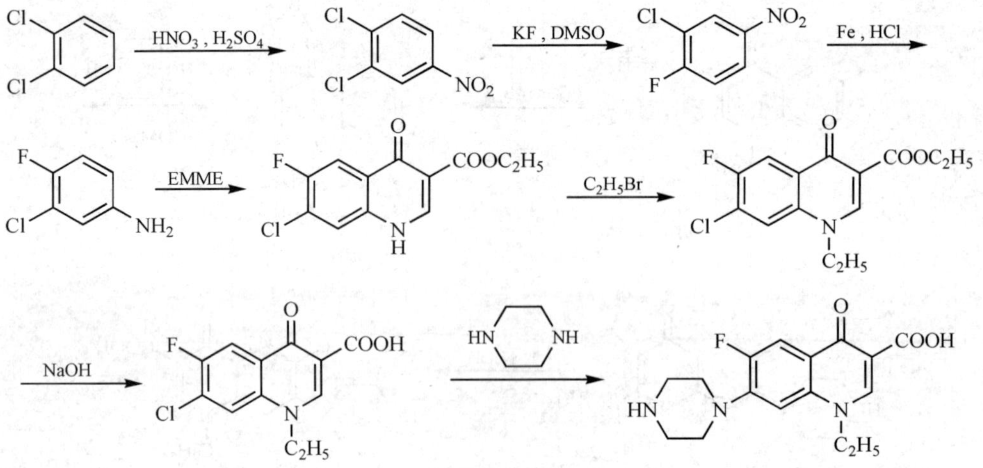

Route 2：

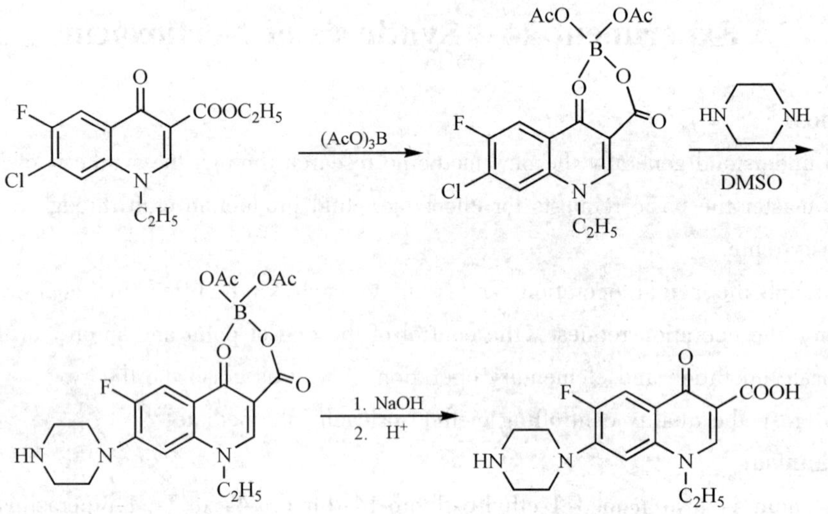

一、4-氟-3-氯-硝基苯的合成

【目的要求】

1. 掌握硝化反应的基本操作。
2. 了解氟化反应的原理并掌握其基本操作。

【实验原理】

反应式：

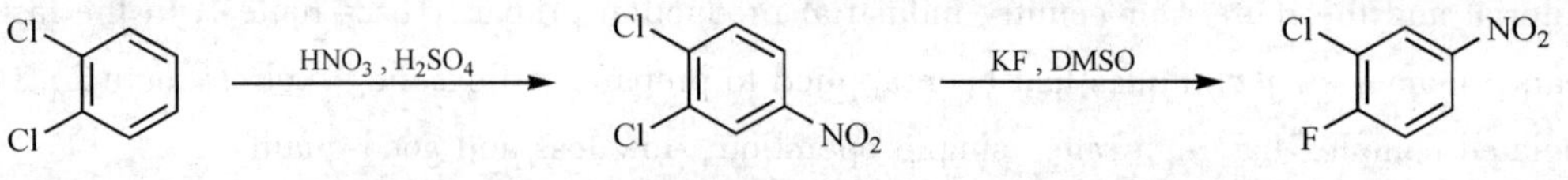

【实验方法】

（一）3,4-二氯硝基苯的制备

在装有搅拌器、回流冷凝器、温度计、滴液漏斗的四颈瓶中，先加入硝酸 51 g，水浴冷却下，滴加硫酸 79 g，控制滴加速度，使温度保持在 50℃以下。滴加完毕，换滴液漏斗，于 40℃～50℃内滴加邻二氯苯 35 g，40 min 内滴完，升温至 60℃，反应 2 h，静置分层，取上层油状液体倾入 5 倍量水中，搅拌，固化，放置 30 min，过滤，水洗至 pH 6～7，真空干燥，称重，计算收率。

（二）4-氟-3-氯-硝基苯的合成

在装有搅拌器、回流冷凝器、温度计、氯化钙干燥管的四颈瓶中，加入 3,4-二氯硝基苯 40 g、无水二甲亚砜 73 g、无水氟化钾 23 g，升温到回流温度 194℃～198℃，在此温度下快速搅拌 1～1.5 h，冷却至 50℃左右，加入 75 ml 水，充分搅拌，倒入分液漏斗中，静置分层，分出下层油状物。安装水蒸气蒸馏装置，进行水蒸气蒸馏，得淡黄色固体，过滤，水洗至中性，真空干燥，得 4-氟-3-氯-硝基苯。

［注释］

1. 第一步反应是混酸硝化。硫酸可以防止副反应的进行，并可以增加被硝化物的溶解度；硝酸生成 NO^{2+}，是硝化剂。

2. 此硝化反应需达到 40℃才能反应，低于此温度，滴加混酸会导致大量混酸聚集，一旦反应引发，聚集的混酸会使反应温度急剧升高，生成许多副产物，因此滴加混酸时应调节滴加速度，控制反应温度在 40℃～50℃。

3. 上述方法所得的产品纯度已经足够用于下步反应，如要得到较纯的产品，可以采用水蒸气蒸馏或减压蒸馏的方法。

4. 3,4-二氯硝基苯的 mp. 39℃～41℃，不能用红外灯或烘箱干燥。

5. 第二步的氟化反应为绝对无水反应，一切仪器及药品必须绝对无水，微量水会导致收率大幅下降。

6. 为保证反应液的无水状态，可在刚回流时蒸出少量二甲亚砜，将反应液中的微量水分带出。

7. 进行水蒸气蒸馏时，少量冷凝水就已足够，大量冷凝水会导致 4-氟-3-氯-硝基苯固化，堵塞冷凝管。

【思考题】

1. 硝化试剂有许多种，请举出其中几种并说明其各自的特点。

2. 配制混酸是能否将浓硝酸加到浓硫酸中去？为什么？

3. 如何检查反应是否已进行完全？

4. 请指出提高第二步氟化反应收率的关键是什么。如果延长反应时间会得到什么样的结果？

5. 水溶液中的二甲亚砜如何回收？

Ⅰ. Preparation of 4-fluoro-3-chloronitrobenzene

Purpose

1. To master the basic operation ofnitrification reaction
2. To learn the principle of the fluorination reaction and master the basic operation.

Mechanism

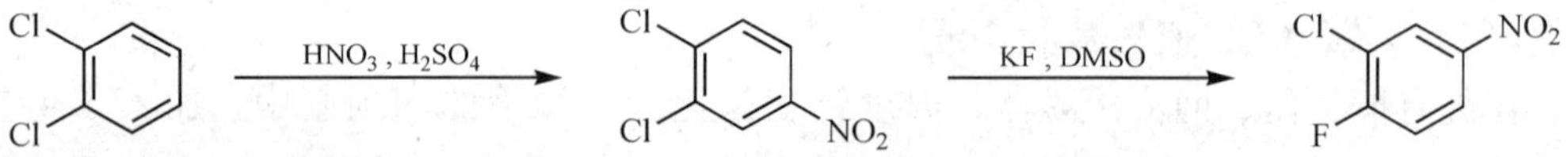

Experiment method

1. Preparation of 3,4-dichloronitrobenzene

In a four-necked flask equipped with an efficient mercury-sealed stirrer, a dropping funnel, a thermometer, and a reflux condenser, the mixture solution of 51 g of nitric acid and 79 g of sulfuric acid is added from a dropping funnel with water cooling at such a rate that the internal temperature always remains at below 50℃. Then, 35 g of 1,2-dichlorobenzene is also added from another funnel cooling at such a rate that the internal temperature always remains at about 40-50℃(during about 40 min). After that, raise the temperature a little to 60℃, and continue stirring at this temperature for 2 hours. Then, the organic layer is carefully poured into about five of its volume water, formation of a solid mass of crystals needs about 30 minutes. Filter and ish with water until the pH of the filtrate reaches about 6-7, then, dried under vacuum. Calculate the yield.

2. Preparation of 4-fluoro-3-chloronitrobenzene

In a four-necked flask with an efficient mercury-sealed stirrer, a thermometer, and a reflux condenser fitted with a calcium chloride tube, place 40 g of 3,4-dichloride, 73 g of thinly chloride anhydrous, and potassium fluoride, raise the temperature to 194-198℃. The mixture is allowed to stand at this temperature for 1 to 1.5 hours with stirring, after cooling to 50℃, then, add 75 ml of water. The organic layer is separated into the separating funnel. The light yellow solid is formed when the organic layer is distilled with water. Filter and ish it with water until the pH of the filtrate reaches 7, then dried under reduced pressure.

Notes:

(1) The first step reaction is nitrification with the nitrosulfuric acid. The sulfuric acid may prevent by-products from being produced, and may increase the solubility of nitration. The nitric acid produces NO_2^+, which is the nitrating agent.

(2) This nitration must achieve 40℃. If lower than this temperature, dropping the nitrosulfuric acid will cause the massive nitrosulfuric acid to gather, which results in high temperature and many by-products. Therefore the speed of dropping nitrosulfuric acid should be controlled to retain the temperature at 40-50℃.

（3） The purity of the product obtained from above method is enough for the next step. It can also be distilled with steam or under reduced pressure to get purer product.

（4） 3,4-dichloronitrobenzene mp. 39-41℃， cannot be dried under infra – red lamp or oven

（5） The fluorination reaction must be absolutely anhydrous including all instruments and drugs， the micro water will cause the yield drop largely.

（6） In order to guarantee anhydrous condition， distill off a few thionyl chloride when just reflux so that the micro water can be carried off.

（7） A little condensed water is enough when distill with steam， large amount will solidify the 4-fluro-3-chloronitrobeneze.

Questions

1. There are many kinds of nitration reagents， please point out several kinds and explain its respective characteristics.

2. Whether is the nitric acid added into the sulfuric acid? Why?

3. How to examine whether the reaction goes on completely?

4. Please point out the key to enhance the yield of the fluorination reaction. What will be obtained if prolong the reaction time?

5. How to recycle thionyl chloride in water solution?

二、4-氟-3-氯-苯胺的制备

【目的要求】

熟悉硝基还原反应的原理并掌握其基本操作。

【实验原理】

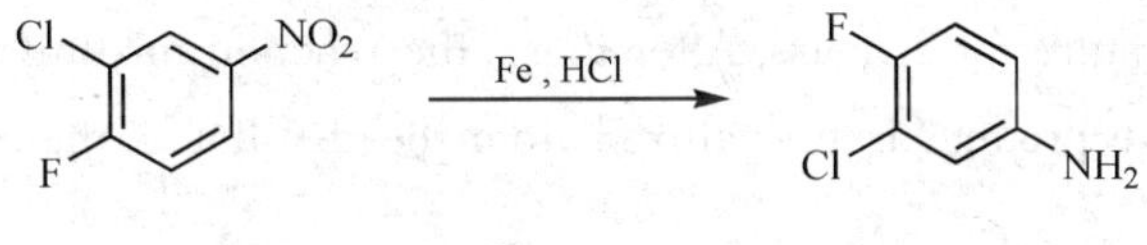

【实验方法】

在装有搅拌、回流冷凝器、温度计的三颈瓶中投入铁粉51.5 g、水173 ml、氯化钠4.3 g、浓盐酸2 ml，搅拌下于100℃活化10 min，降温至85℃，在快速搅拌下，先加入4-氟-3-氯-硝基苯15 g，温度自然升至95℃，10 min后再加入4-氟-3-氯-硝基苯15 g，于95℃反应2 h，然后将反应液进行水蒸气蒸馏，馏出液中加入冰，使产品固化完全，过滤，于30℃下干燥，得4-氟-3-氯-苯胺，mp. 44℃ ~47℃。

［注释］

1. 胺的制备通常是在盐酸或醋酸存在下用铁粉还原硝基化合物而制得。该法原料便宜，操作简便，收率稳定，适于工业生产。

2. 铁粉由于表面上有氧化铁膜，需经活化才能反应，铁粉粗细一般以60目为宜。

3. 由于铁粉密度较大，搅拌速度慢则不能将铁粉搅匀，会在烧瓶下部结块，影响收率，因此该反应应剧烈搅拌。

4. 水蒸气蒸馏应控制冷凝水的流速，防止4-氟-3-氯-苯胺固化，堵塞冷凝管。

5. 4-氟-3-氯-苯胺的熔点低（40℃～43℃），故应低温干燥。

【思考题】

1. 此反应用的铁粉为硅铁粉，含有部分硅，如用纯铁粉效果如何？
2. 试举出其他还原硝基化合物成胺的还原剂，并简述各自特点。
3. 对于这步反应如何检测其反应终点？
4. 反应中为何分步投料？

Ⅱ. Preparation of EMME

Purpose

To understand generally the principle of the nitro reduction and master the basic operation.

Mechanism

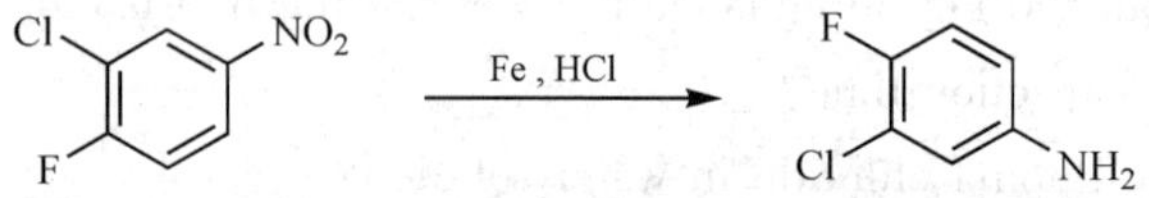

Experiment method

A mixture of 51.5 g of iron, 71ml of water, 2 ml of the concentrated hydrochloric acid are placed into a three-necked flask, and the flask is fitted with an efficient mercury-sealed stirrer, a thermometer, and a reflux condenser. Stir the mixture for ten mins at 100℃, add 15 g of the 4-fluoro-3-chloronitrobenzene, then raise the temperature to 95℃, and continue stirring at this temperature for 2 hours. After that, the reaction mixture is distilled with water, after ice is added, the product is crystallized from the distillate, then filter and dried under 35℃.

Notes:

(1) The amine is usually prepared by using iron dust to reduce the nitro compounds when hydrochloric acid or the acetic acid exists. The method has advantages of cheap material, simple operation, stable yield and is also suitable for the industrial production.

(2) Because the iron dust has iron membrane on the surface. It must be activated before hand. The granularity of the powdered iron is generally 60 item.

(3) Because of the high density of iron dust, the stirring speed should be fierce. Otherwise it cannot mix the iron dust evenly, further agglomerate lower part of flask, influence the yield.

(4) The speed of cooling water should be controlled during steam distillation in order to prevent 4-fluoro-3-chloroaniline from being solidified, and further jaming the condenser.

(5) 4-fluoro-3-chloroaniline melting point is low (40 – 43℃), therefore it should be

dried at low temperature.

Questions

1. The iron powder in this reaction contains partial silicon, what will be the effect if the pure iron dust is used?

2. Please give other reducing agent which can reduce nitro compound to amine and summarize the characteristic respectively.

3. How to examine the end point?

4. Why place the materials in different time?

三、7-氯-6-氟-1,4-二氢-4-氧喹啉-3-羧酸乙酯（环合物）的制备

【目的要求】

1. 了解制备 EMME 的缩合反应和 Could-Jacobs 反应的机理。

2. 掌握制备 EMME 和 Could Jacobs 反应的基本操作。

【实验原理】

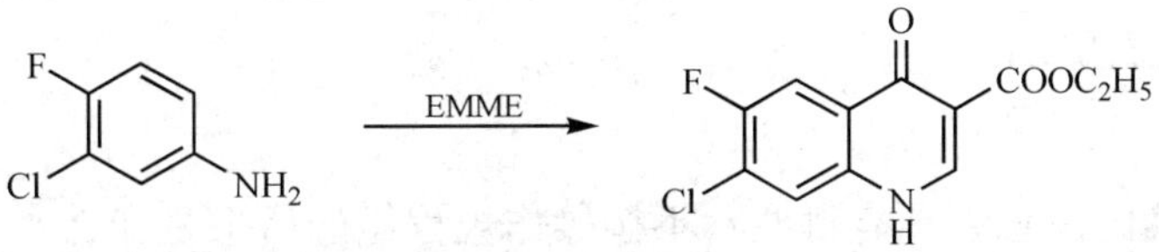

该环合反应是典型的 Could-Jacobs 反应，考虑苯环上的取代基的定位效应及空间效应，3-位氯的对位远比邻位活泼，但也不能忽略邻位的取代。反应条件控制不当，便会按下式反应形成反环物：

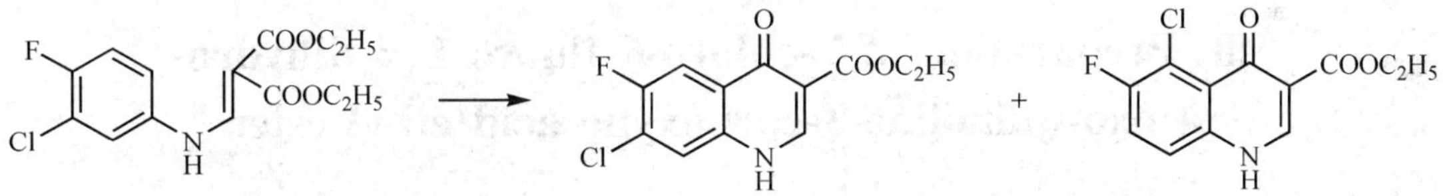

【实验方法】

（一）乙氧基次甲基丙二酸二乙酯（EMME）的制备

在装有搅拌器、温度计、滴液漏斗、蒸馏装置的四颈瓶中，加入原甲酸三乙酯78 g，$ZnCl_2$ 0.1 g，搅拌，加热，升温至 120℃，蒸出乙醇，降温至 70℃，于 70℃～80℃内滴加第二批原甲酸三乙酯 20 g 及醋酐 6 g，于 0.5 h 内滴完，然后升温到 152℃～156℃，保温反应2 h。冷却至室温，将反应液倾入圆底烧瓶中，水泵减压回收原甲酸三乙酯（bp. 140℃，70℃ / 5333 Pa）。冷到室温，换油泵进行减压蒸馏，收集 120℃～140℃ / 666.6 Pa 的馏分，得乙氧基次甲基丙二酸二乙酯。

（二）7-氯-6-氟-1,4-二氢-4-氧喹啉-3-羧酸乙酯（环合物）的制备

在装有搅拌器、回流冷凝器、温度计的三颈瓶中分别投入 4-氟-3-氯－苯胺15 g、EMME 24 g，快速搅拌下加热到 120℃，于 120℃～130℃反应 2 h。放冷至室温，将回流装置改成蒸馏装置，加入石蜡油 80 ml，加热到 260℃～270℃，有大量乙醇生成，回

收乙醇反应 30 min 后，冷却到 60℃以下，过滤，滤饼分别用甲苯、丙酮洗至灰白色，干燥，测熔点，mp. 297℃ ~298℃，计算收率。

[注释] 1. 第一步反应是一缩合反应，$ZnCl_2$是 Lewis 酸，作为催化剂。

2. 减压蒸馏所需真空度要达 666.6 Pa 以上，才可进行蒸馏操作，真空度小，蒸馏温度高，导致收率下降。

3. 减压回收原甲酸三乙酯时亦可进行常压蒸馏，收集 140℃ ~150℃的沸点馏分。蒸出的原甲酸三乙酯可以套用。

4. 第二步反应为无水反应，所有仪器应干燥，严格按无水反应操作进行，否则会导致 EMME 分解。

5. 环合反应温度控制在 260℃ ~270℃，为避免温度超过 270℃，可在将要达到 270℃时缓慢加热。反应开始后，反应液变黏稠，为避免局部过热，应快速搅拌。

6. 为减少反环物的生成，应注意以下几点：a. 反应温度低，有利于反环物的生成。因此，反应温度应快速达到 260℃，且保持在 260℃ ~270℃。b. 加大溶剂用量可以降低反环物的生成。从经济的角度来讲，采用溶剂与反应物用量比为 3∶1 时比较合适。c. 用二甲苯或二苯砜为溶剂时，会减少反环物的生成，但价格昂贵。亦可用廉价的工业柴油代替石蜡油。

【思考题】

1. 减压蒸馏的注意事项有哪些？不按操作规程做的后果是什么？
2. 第一步反应所用的 Lewis 酸除 $ZnCl_2$外，还有哪些可以替代？
3. 请写出 Could-Jacobs 反应历程，并讨论何种反应条件有利于提高反应收率。
4. 该反应为高温反应，试举出几种高温浴装置，并写出安全注意事项。

Ⅲ. Preparation of 7-chloro-6-fluoro-1,4-dihydro-4-oxo-quinoline-3-carboxylic acid ethyl ester

Purpose

1. To learn the mechanism of the condensation reaction and the Could-Jacobs reation.
2. To master the basic operation of the two reactions.

Mechanism

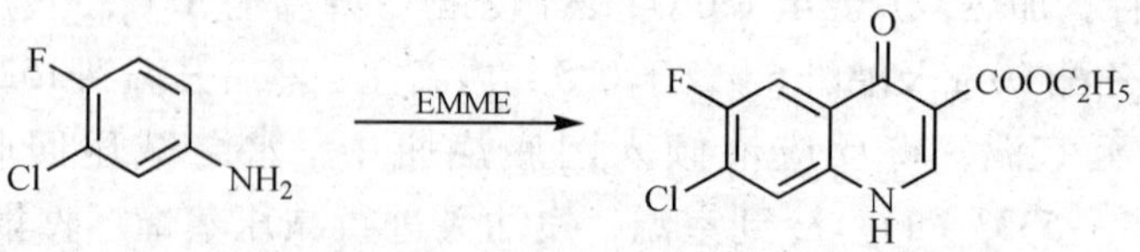

The cyclization is typical Could-Jacobs reaction. Considering localization and the steric effect of substitution on the benzene ring, the substitution of 3-chlorine is far more active than ortho-position, but cannot neglect the substitution ortho-position. If the condition control is improper, then the counter-link can be produced:

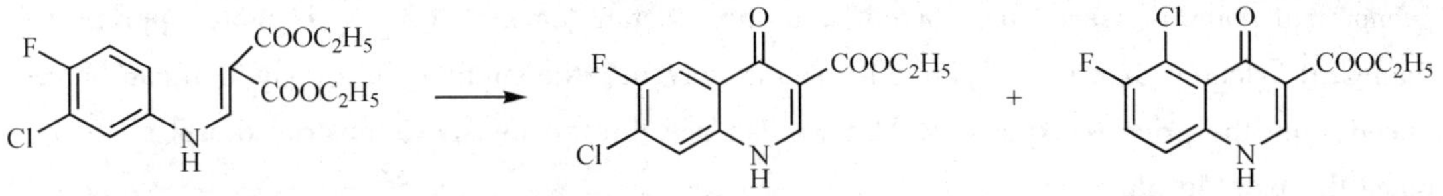

Experiment method

1. Preparation of EMME

In a four-necked flask with an efficient mercury-sealed stirrer, a dropping funnel, a thermometer and a reflux condenser, place 78 g of the triethylformate, and 0.1 g of znic chloride, raise the temperature to 120℃ under stirring. Distill alcohol, low the temperature to 70℃, place 20 g of triethylformate, 6 g of acetic anhydride acid is added from a dropping funnel with water cooling at such a rate that the internal temperature always remains at 60-70℃. After that, raise the temperature to 152-156℃, the mixture is allowed to stand at this temperature for 2 hours. After cooling to the room temperature, the reaction solution is carefully poured into the round-bottomed flask, it is distilled under vacuum with a water pump, b.p 70℃/5333Pa. Then cooling to room temperature, the residue is distilled under reduce pressure with an oil pump, b.p 120-140℃/666.6Pa.

2. Preparation of 7-chloro-6-fluoro-1, 4-dihydro-4-oxo-quinoline-3-carboxylic acid ethyl ester

In a three-necked flask with an efficient mercury-sealed stirrer, a thermometer, and a reflux condenser, place 15 g of 4-floro-3-chloroaniline and 24 g of EMEA, raise the temperature to 120℃ under rapidly stirring, continue stirring at the temperature 120 -130℃ for 2 h. Cool to r. t. and place 80 ml of paraffin oil, heat up to 260-270℃, distill alcohol, 30 minutes later, low the temperature to 60℃, filter, ished with xyene, acetone, dry, measure the mp (297-298℃) and calculate the yield.

Notes:

(1) The first reaction is a condensation reaction, $ZnCl_2$ is Lewis acid as a catalyst.

(2) The vacuum degree has to reach above 666.6 Pa, or it will make the yield dropping.

(3) The triethylformate can also be distilled under normal pressure, collect distillate at 140-150℃. The triethylformate can be recycled.

(4) This second reaction should be anhydrous, and all instruments should be dry, otherwise EMME would be decomposed.

(5) The temperature of cyclization should be controlled at 260-270℃, slowly heat up when the temperature is going to achieve 270℃. The mixture becomes thick, stir fast in order to avoid partial heating.

(6) In order to reduce the counter-link production, the following several points should be paid attention to: A. The low reaction temperature is advantageous to the counter-link production. Therefore, the reaction temperature should fast achieve 260℃, also maintain at 260-270℃. B. Enlarging the solvent amount may reduce the counter-link production. From the

economical point of view, the solvent and the reactant amount (3/1) is more appropriate than C. If xylene or benzoin sulphone is used as solvent, the counter-link production can be reduced, but the price is expensive. Also we can use the inexpensive industrial diesel oil to replace the paraffin oil.

Questions

1. What should we pay attention to when distilling under reduced pressure. What will be the result if not operate according to the instruction?

2. Except for the $ZnCl_2$, which lewis acid can be used in the first reaction?

3. Please write the Could-Jacobs mechanism of reaction, and discuss which condition is more advantageous to enhance the yield.

4. This reaction needs high temperature, try to point out several high temperature baths installment, and write the attentive matters on safety.

四、1-乙基-7-氯-6-氟-1,4-二氢-4-氧喹啉-3-羧酸乙酯（乙基物）制备

【目的要求】

掌握乙基化反应的原理和操作。

【实验原理】

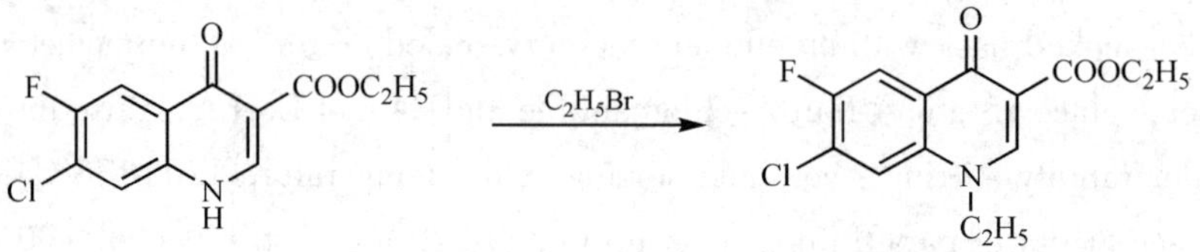

【实验方法】

在装有搅拌器、回流冷凝器、温度计、滴液漏斗的250 ml四颈瓶中，加入环合物25 g、无水碳酸钾30.8 g、DMF 125 g，搅拌，加热到70℃，于70℃～80℃下，在40～60 min内滴加溴乙烷25 g。滴加完毕，升温至100℃～110℃，保温反应6～8 h，反应完毕，减压回收70%～80%的DMF，降温至50℃左右，加入200 ml水，析出固体，过滤，水洗，干燥，得粗品，用乙醇重结晶。

[**注释**] 1. 反应中所用DMF要预先进行干燥，少量水分对收率有很大影响，所用无水碳酸钾需炒过。

2. 溴乙烷沸点低，易挥发，为避免损失，可将滴液漏斗的滴管加长，插到液面以下，同时注意反应装置的密闭性。

3. 反应液加水是要降至50℃左右，温度太高导致酯键水解，过低会使产物结块，不易处理。

4. 环合物在溶液中酮式与烯醇式有一平衡，反应后可得到少量乙基化合物，该化合物随主产物一起进入后续反应，使生成6-氟-1,4-二氢-4-氧代7-(1-哌嗪基)喹啉（简称脱羧物），成为氟哌酸中的主要杂质。不同的乙基化试剂，*O*-乙基产物生成量不一

样，采用 BrEt 时较低。

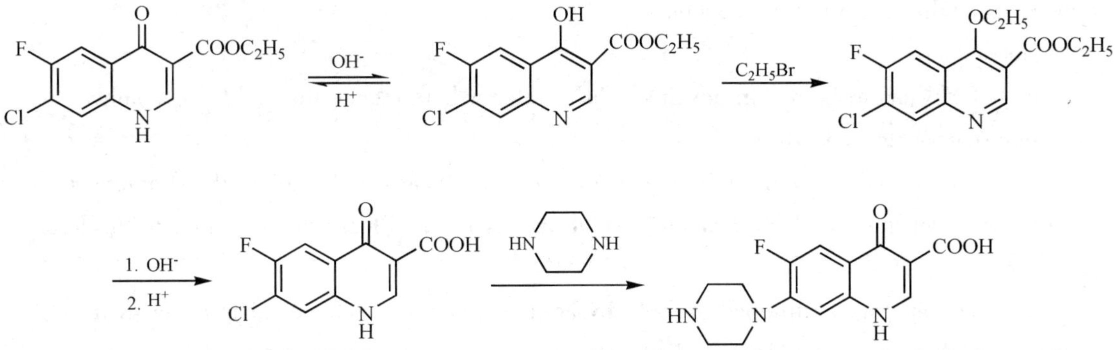

5. 滤饼洗涤时要将颗粒碾细，同时用大量水冲洗，否则会有少量 K_2CO_3残留。

6. 乙醇重结晶操作过程：取粗品，加入 4 倍量的乙醇，加热至沸，溶解。稍冷，加入活性炭，回流 10 min，趁热过滤，滤液冷却至 10℃结晶析出，过滤，洗涤，干燥，得精品，测熔点（mp. 144℃ ~ 145℃）。母液中尚有部分产品，可以浓缩一半体积后，冷却，析晶，所得产品亦可用于下步投料。

【思考题】

1. 对于该反应，请找出其他的乙基化试剂，略述优缺点。
2. 该反应的副产物是什么？简述减少副产物的方法。
3. 采用何种方法可使溴乙烷得到充分合理的利用？
4. 如减压回收 DMF 后不降温，加水稀释，对反应有何影响？

Ⅳ. Preparation of 1-ethyl-7-chloro-6-fluoro-1,4-dihydro-4-oxo-quinolone-3-carboxylic acid ethyl ester

Purpose

To master the basic principle and operation of ethylation reaction.

Mechanism

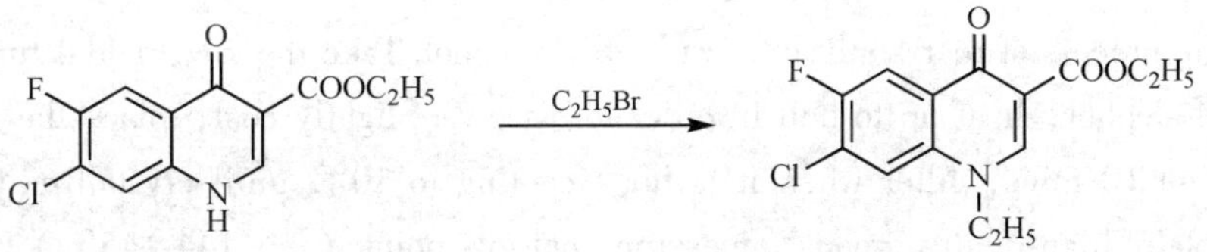

Experiment method

In a 250ml four-necked flask equipped with an efficient mercury-sealed stirrer, a dropping funnel, a thermometer, and a reflux condenser, place 25 g of cyclization, 30 g of anhydrous potassium carbonate, 125 g of DMF, raise the temperature to 70℃. Drop ethyl bromide in 40-60 mins at 70-80℃, then, raise the temperature to 100-110℃, continue for 6-8h. Distill DMF, cool to 50℃, then, the organic layer is added 20ml of water. After the formation of a solid mass of crystals, filter, ished with water, dried, the raw product is obtained, crystallized with ethyl alcohol.

Notes:

(1) DMF has to be dry in advance. Little water will influence the yield, and anhydrous potassium carbonate needs to fry.

(2) Boiling point of ethyl bromide is low, easy to volatilize. Lengthen the dropping funnel dropper, set the liquid level below, which avoids losing. Please pay attention to the leak-proofness

(3) The mixture is dropped to 50℃ by adding water. The ester bond is made hydrolysis under too high temperature. The product can cause to agglomerate under too low temperature and is difficult to process.

(4) The cyclization has a balance between the ketonic and the enol form in the solution, may obtain a few ethyl compound, which companies the main product entering the next step, and produce 6-fluoro-4-oxo-7-piperazin-1-yl-1, 4-dihydro-quinoline-3-carboxylic acid, which becomes the main impurity. Different ethylic reagent, the quantity of *O*-ethyl product is different. BrEt is low relatively.

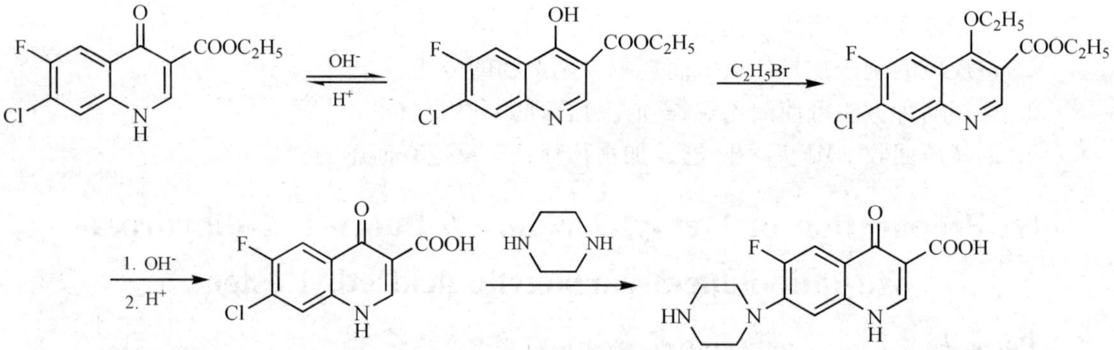

(5) When ish the cake, the pellet should be made thin, at the same time massive water flushing, otherwise a few K_2CO_3 will remain.

(6) The process of recrystallization with ethyl alcohol. Take the raw, add 4 times of quantities of ethyl alcohol, heat up to boil in order to dissolve. Slightly cool, place the active charcoal, reflux for 10 mins, filter when it is hot, cooling to 10℃ until crystallize. Filter, ish, dry, and obtain high-quality goods, measure melting point (mp. 144-145℃). Concentrate the mother liquor to a half-volume, cool, the obtained product also might be used in next step.

Questions

1. Regarding to this reaction, please find out other ethylic reagents, give the advantages and shortcomings in brief.

2. What is the by-product in this reaction? Summarize methods how to reduce the by – product.

3. How to make full use of ethyl bromide ?

4. After recycling DMF under reduced pressure, if not decrease temperature, but thin up, what will happen about the reaction?

五、诺氟沙星的制备（一）

【目的要求】

了解 *N*-烷基化反应的基本原理并掌握制备诺氟沙星相关实验操作。

【实验原理】

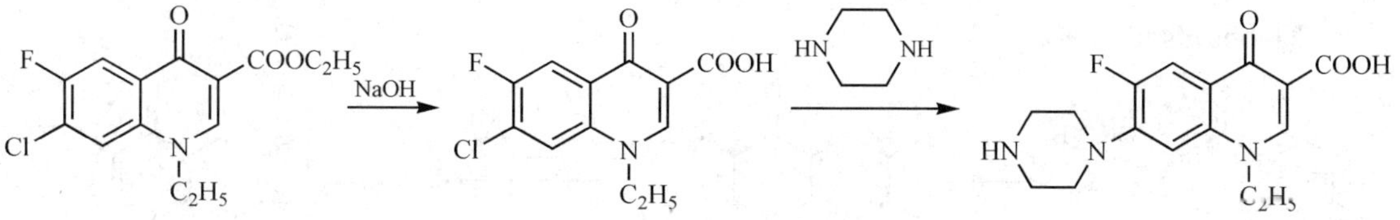

【实验方法】

1. 1-乙基-7-氯-6-氟-1,4-二氢-4-氧喹啉-3-羧酸（水解物）的制备

在装有搅拌器、冷凝器、温度计的三颈瓶中，加入 20 g 乙基物以及碱液（由氢氧化钠 5. 5 g 和蒸馏水 75 g 配成），加热至 95℃ ~100℃，保温反应 10 min。冷却至 50℃，加入水 125 ml 稀释，浓盐酸调 pH 6，冷却至 20℃，过滤，水洗，干燥，测熔点（若熔点低于 270℃，需进行重结晶），计算收率。

2. 诺氟沙星的制备

在装有搅拌器、回流冷凝器、温度计的 150 ml 三颈瓶中，投入水解物 10 g、无水哌嗪 13 g、吡啶 65 g，回流反应 6 h，冷却到 10℃，析出固体，抽滤，干燥，称重，测熔点，mp. 215℃ ~218℃。

将上述粗品加入 100 ml 水溶解，用冰醋酸调 pH 7，抽滤，得精品，干燥，称重，测熔点，mp. 216℃ ~220℃，计算收率和总收率。

［**注释**］1. 在第一步中，由于反应物不溶于碱，而产品溶于碱，反应完全后，反应液澄清。

2. 在调 pH 之前应先粗略计算盐酸用量，快到终点时，将盐酸稀释，以防加入过量的酸。

3. 重结晶的方法：取粗品，加入 5 倍量上步回收的 DMF，加热溶解，加入活性炭，再加热，过滤，除去活性炭，冷却，结晶，过滤，洗涤，干燥，得精品。

3. 第二步反应为氮烃化反应，注意温度与时间对反应的影响。

4. 反应物的 6 位氟亦可与 7 位氯竞争性地参与反应，会有诺氟沙星副产物生成，最多可达 25%。

【思考题】

1. 水解反应的副产物有几种，带入下一步会有何后果？

2. 浓盐酸调 pH 值快到 6 时，溶液会有何变化？为什么？

3. 第二步反应中吡啶有哪些作用，并指出该反应的优缺点。
4. 用水重结晶主要分离什么杂质？设计出几种其他的精制方法，并与该法比较。
5. 通过本实验编制一份工艺操作规程及工艺流程，并对本工艺路线作一评价。
6. 做一张本产品的红外光谱及核磁共振氢谱图，并进行解析。

V. Preparation of Norfloxacin

Purpose

To learn the mechanism of nitrogen alkylation and master the operation of Norfloxacin.

Mechanism

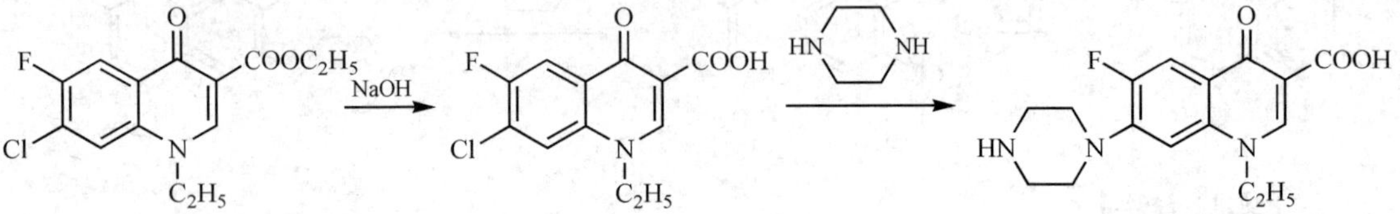

Experiment method

1. Preparation of 1-ethyl-7-chloro-6-fluoro-1, 4-dihydro-4-oxo-quinoline-3-carboxylic acid ethyl ester

In a three-necked flask with an efficient mercury-sealed stirrer, a thermometer, and a reflux condenser, place 20 g of ethide, and alkali solution (formed of 5. 5 g of NaOH and 75 g of water), raise the temperature to 95-100℃ , continue stirring at the temperature for 10 mins, cool to 50℃. Dilute with 125ml of water, The pH is adjusted to 6 with HCl, low the temperature to 20℃ , filter, ish with water, dry, measure the mp (if below 270℃ , crystallization again), calculate the yield.

3. Preparation of Norfloxacin

In a three-necked flask with an efficient mercury-sealed stirrer, a thermometer, and a reflux condenser, 10 g of hydrolysate, 10 g of anhydrous piperazine and 65g of pyridine are placed. Raise the temperature to reflux for 6 h, cool to 10℃ , then the solid is formed, filter, dry, weigh, measure mp. (215-218℃) .

The raw above is dissolved with 125ml of water. The pH is adjusted to 7 with glacial acetic acid, filter, dry, weigh, measure the mp. (216-220℃), calculate the yield and total yield.

Notes:

(1) Because the reactant does not dissolve in alkali, but the product dissolves in the alkali. The reaction fluid will be clear if it is over.

(2) Before adjusting pH, first to calculate the amount. When approximate to the end point, dilute the hydrochloric acid in case of excessive acid.

(3) Recrystallization method: Take the raw, 5 times the recycling DMF is added, heat up to dissolve and add the activated carbon. Heat again, filter activated carbon off , cool, fil-

ter the crystallization, ish, dry and obtain high - quality product.

(4) This second step is nitrogen alkylation, pay attention to the influence of temperature and time.

(5) The reactant 6-fluoro may compete with 7-chloro, which produces the by-product, most may reach 25%.

Questions

1. In the first step, there are several kinds of by - products, what will it cause if the by-product is brought into next step?

2. What will happen in solution when pH is adjusted to 6 with concentrated hydrochloric acid? Why?

3. What does the pyridine act in the second step? And point out the advantages and shortcomings.

4. What impurity is mainly separated through the recrystallization by water? Design other methods to purify the product and compare it with this method.

5. Establish a working instruction and the technical process according to this experiment, and make an appraisal on this craft route.

6. Make the infrared spectrum and the nuclear magnetic resonance hydrogen spectrogram, and analysize.

六、硼螯合物的制备

【目的要求】

熟悉硼螯合物的制备原理并掌握实验方法。

【实验原理】

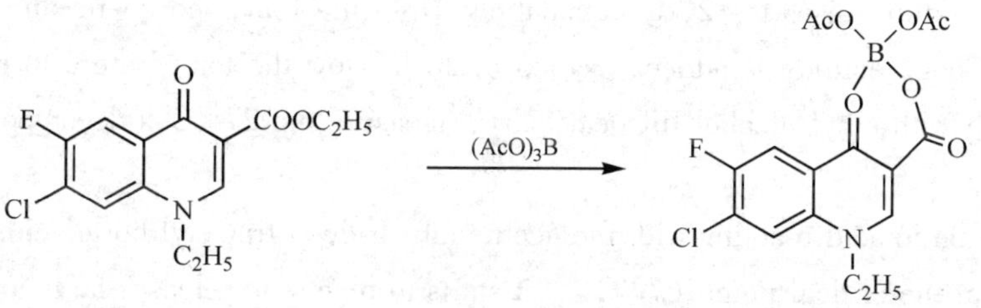

【实验方法】

在装有搅拌器、冷凝器、温度计、滴液漏斗的250 ml四颈瓶中，加入氯化锌、硼酸3.3 g及少量醋酐（醋酐总计用量为17 g），搅拌，加热至79℃，反应引发后，停止加热，自动升温至120℃。滴加剩余醋酐，加完后回流1 h，冷却，加入乙基物10 g，回流2.5 h，冷却到室温，加水，过滤，少量冰乙醇洗至灰白色，干燥，测熔点，mp. 275℃（分解）。

［注释］1. 硼酸与醋酐反应生成硼酸三乙酰酯，此反应到达79℃临界点时才开始反应，并释放出大量热，温度急剧升高。如果量大，则有冲料的危险，建议采用250

ml 以上的反应瓶，并缓慢加热。

2. 由于螯合物在乙醇中有一定溶解度，为避免产品损失，最后洗涤时，可先用冰水洗涤，温度降下来后，再用冰乙醇洗涤。

【思考题】

1. 搅拌快慢对该反应有何影响?

2. 加入乙基物后，反应体系中主要有那几种物质?

Ⅵ. Preparation of boron chelated complex

Purpose

To learn the principle of the boron chelated complex operation and master the experiment method.

Mechanism

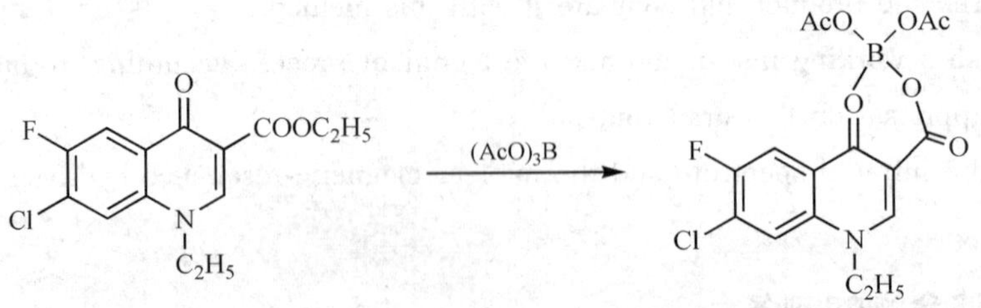

Experiment method

In a 250ml four-necked flask equipped with an efficient mercury-sealed stirrer, a dropping funnel, a thermometer, and a reflux condenser, $ZnCl_2$ boric acid, 3. 3 g of acetic anhydride (total: 17 g) are placed. Raise the temperature to 79℃. Once start to react, stop heating, temperature raises to 120℃ automaticly. Drop the remained acetic anhydride, then, reflux for 1h. Cool, enthide is added, reflux for 20 h, low the temperature to r. t. , add water, filter, ish with ethyl alcohol till peal, dry, measure mp 275℃ (decompose).

Notes:

(1) The boric acid reacting with the acetic anhydride is triacetyl boric acid. When the reaction arrives at the critical point (79℃), it starts to react and releases large amount of heat, the temperature raises suddenly. The mixture may flush if the quantity is large, so it is suggested that the flask should be above 250 ml and slowly heat up.

(2) Because chelated complex has the certain solubility in ethyl alcohol, in order to avoid being losed, first to ish it with ice, cool down and ish it with ethyl alcohol.

Questions

1. What is the influence caused by the speed of stir in this reaction?

2. What kind of matter is main in the reacting system after adding the ethylation?

七、诺氟沙星的制备（二）

【目的要求】

掌握诺氟沙星的第二种制备方法。

【实验原理】

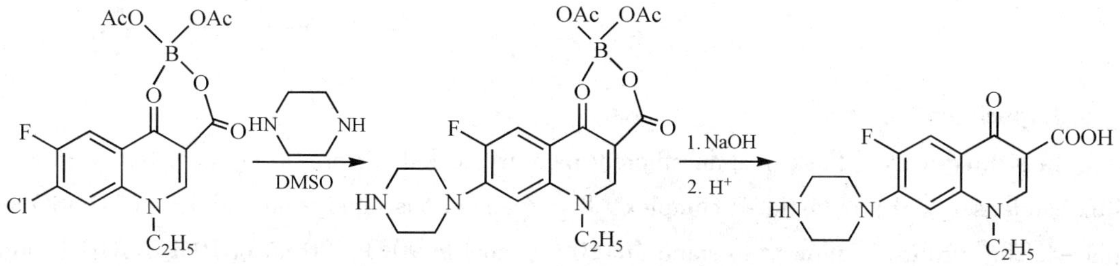

【实验方法】

在装有搅拌器、回流冷凝器、温度计的三颈瓶中，加入螯合物 10 g、无水哌嗪 8 g、二甲亚砜（DMSO）30 g，于 110℃反应 3 h，冷却至 90℃，加入 10% NaOH 20 ml，回流 2 h，冷至室温，加 50 ml 水稀释，用乙酸调 pH 7.2，过滤，水洗，得粗品。在 250 ml 烧杯中加入粗品及 100 ml 水，加热溶解后，冷却，用乙酸调 pH 7，析出固体，抽滤，水洗，干燥，得氟哌酸，测熔点，mp. 216℃ ~220℃。

［注释］1. 硼螯合物可以利用 4 位羰基氧的 p 电子向硼原子轨道转移的特性，增强诱导效应，激活 7 – Cl，钝化 6 – F，从而选择性地提高哌嗪化收率，能彻底的防止氯哌酸的生成。

2. 由于氟哌酸溶于碱，如反应液在加入 NaOH 回流后澄清，表示反应已进行完全。

3. 过滤粗品时，要将滤饼中的乙酸盐洗净，防止带入精制过程，影响产品的质量。

【思考题】

1. 试从收率、操作难易、单耗等方面比较两种合成方法。
2. 从该反应的特点出发，选择几种可以替代 DMSO 的溶剂或溶剂系统。

【结构确证】

1. 红外吸收光谱法、标准物 TLC 对照法。
2. 核磁共振光谱法。

Ⅶ. Preparation of Norfloxacin

Purpose

To master another kind of preparation of Norfloxacin.

Mechanism

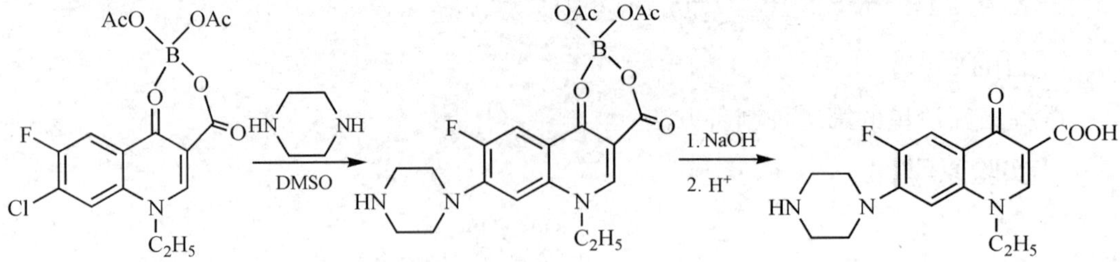

Experiment method

In a three-necked flask with an efficient mercury-sealed stirrer, a thermometer, and a reflux condenser, 20 g of chelated complex, 8 g of anhydrous piperazine and 30 g of DMSO are placed. The mixture is allowed to stand at 110℃, cool to 90℃, 20 ml of 10% NaOH is added, reflux for 2h, cool to rt. Dilute with 50 ml of water, it is adjusted to pH 7. 2 with acetic acid, filter, ish with water to obtain the raw. Place the raw and 100 ml of water in a 250 ml beaker, heated to dissolve, cool. The pH is adjusted to 7 with acetic acid, solid is formed, filter, ish with water, dry to obtain Norfloxacin, measure the mp (216-220℃).

Notes:

(1) Boron chelated complex uses the characteristic p electrons in 4-ketonic oxygens, enhances inductive effect, activates 7-Cl, deactivates 6-F, thus the yield is enhanced selectively and it prevents Norfloxacin from producing thoroughly.

(2) Norfloxacin dissolves in alkali. If the reaction fluid turns to be clear after NaOH is added, which indicates that the reaction is finished completely.

(3) When filtering the raw, ish out the acetate in the cake in order to not be brought into the process of purify.

Questions

1. Compare the two synthetic methods from yield, operation, decrement and so on.

2. Embarks from the characteristic of reaction, choose several kinds of solvent system that can replace DMSO.

Identification

1. Infrared absorption spectroscopy; TLC counterpoint with standard substance.

2. Nuclear magnetic resonance spectroscopy.

实验二十五 盐酸右丙氧芬中间体的合成

盐酸右丙氧芬（dextropropoxyphene hydrochloride），商品名为达尔丰（Darvon），化学名为(+)-2*S*,3*R*-3-甲基-4-二甲氨基-1,2-二苯基-2-丁醇丙酸酯盐酸盐。

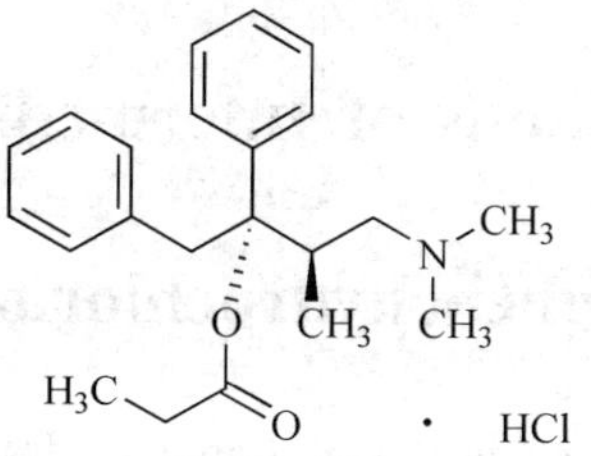

丙氧芬（propoxyphene）含有两个手性碳原子，因此有四个异构体，其中 α-(*d*)-型异构体（2*S*，3*R*）即右氧丙芬可以与阿片 μ 受体结合，具有弱效麻醉镇痛作用，临床上用于缓解轻至中度疼痛。右丙氧芬最早于 1957 年被美国食品药品管理局（FDA）批准在美国上市。在市场上销售的右丙氧芬有其单一制剂（盐酸盐和萘磺酸盐）以及与对乙酰氨基酚等组成的复方制剂（丙氧氨酚复方片）。

后期临床使用中发现，含右丙氧芬的药品制剂存在着严重的心脏毒副作用，且过量服用可危及生命，因此自 2010 年始，右丙氧芬先后在美国、欧洲、中国等多个国家和地区退出市场。

盐酸右丙氧芬的合成路线：

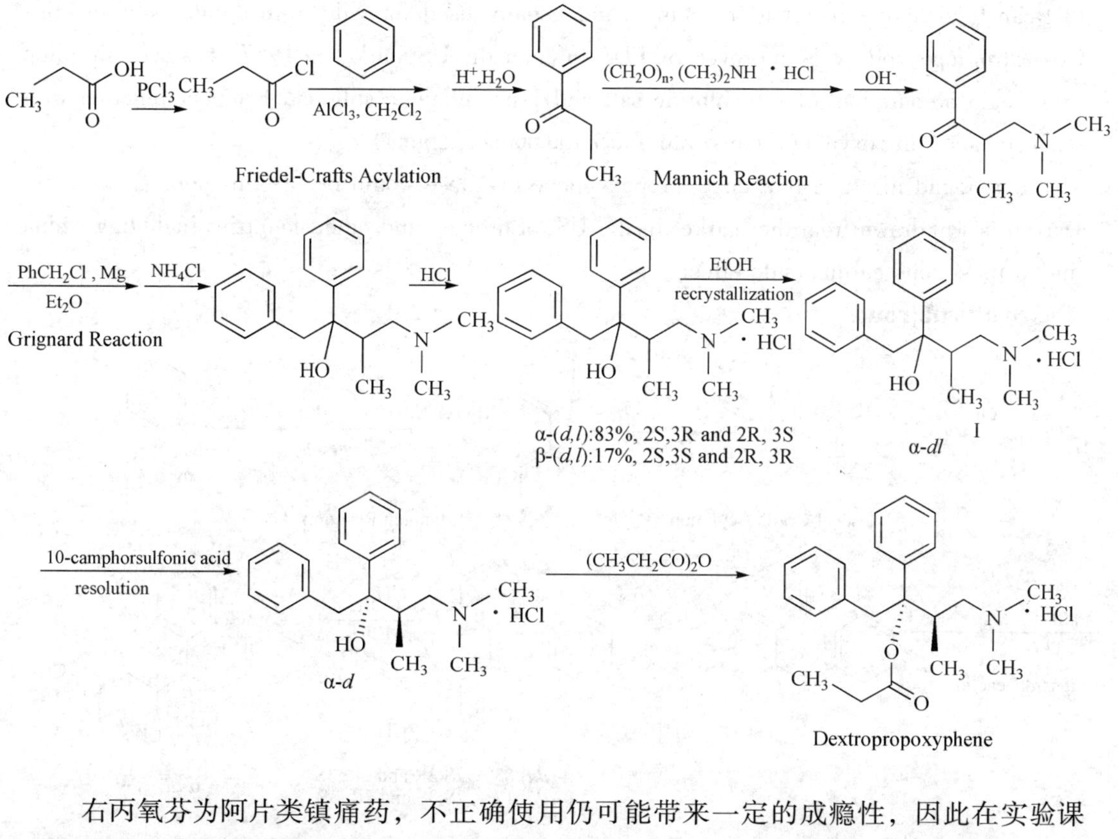

右丙氧芬为阿片类镇痛药，不正确使用仍可能带来一定的成瘾性，因此在实验课的安排中，将合成右丙氧芬的关键中间体 I 即 2*S*，3*R*－3－甲基－4－二甲氨基－1，2－二苯基－2－丁醇作为最终目标产物。通过该中间体的合成，使学生掌握傅－克酰基化反应、曼尼希反应、格氏反应等重要反应的机理和操作步骤，并且熟悉常见的纯化操作如萃取、蒸馏（包括常压和减压）、成盐、重结晶等，提高其实验操作技能。

Experiment 25 Synthesis of Intermediate of Dextropropoxyphenehydrochloride

Dextropropoxyphene hydrochloride (brand name: Darvon; chemical name: (+)-2*S*, 3*R*-4-dimethylamino-3-methyl-1,2-diphenyl-2-butanol propionate).

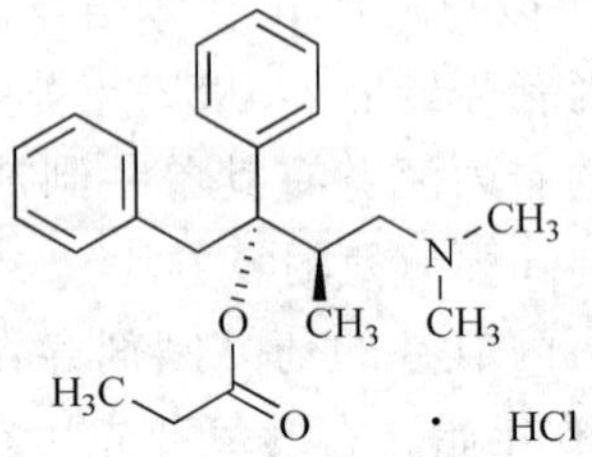

Propoxyphene contains two chiral centers, and therefore four stereoisomers are possible. The α-(*d*)-isomer, namely (2*S*, 3*R*)-dextropropoxyphene, is a weak narcotic analgesic that can bind to the μ-opioid receptor, and usually used for wild-to-moderate pain in clinic. Dextropropoxyphene is approved by FDA to enter the US market in 1957. It is used in clinic in a single preparation (hydrochloride salt and 1-naphthalene sulfonate) or combination with paracetamol (propoxyphene napsylate and paracotamol tablets).

It is found in clinic that dextropropoxyphene overdose would be life-threatening. In 2010, Darvon is withdrawn from the market in the US, Europe, and other countries including China due to its serious cardiac side effect.

Synthetic route

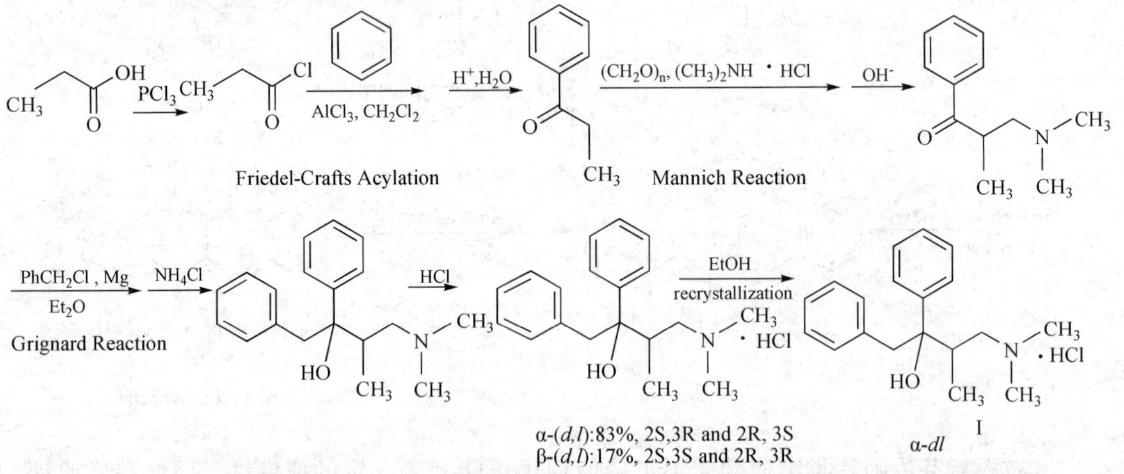

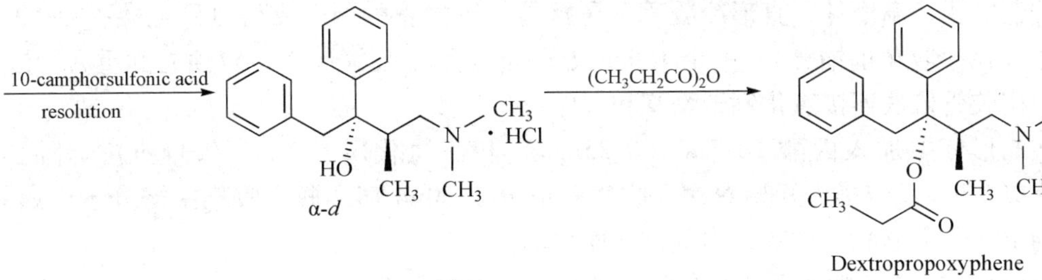

Dextropropoxyphene is an opioid analgesic and its overdose could lead to addiction. Therefore, we take the key intermediate I, 2*S*,3*R*-4-dimethylamino-3-methyl-1,2-diphenyl-2-butanol, as the final target compound. Through the experimental operation, the students will grasp the related mechanisms and processes of reactions including Friedel-Crafts reaction, Mannich reaction, Grignard reaction, and become familiar with the basic purification procedures such as extraction, distillation, salt formation, recrystallization, and so on.

一、丙酰氯的合成

【目的要求】

1. 掌握酰氯的制备方法。
2. 熟悉蒸馏的基本操作。

【实验原理】

酰氯是一种重要的羧酸衍生物，在有机合成、药物合成等方面都有着重要的应用，主要可以发生水解、醇解、氨（胺）解、与有机金属试剂反应、还原反应、α 氢卤化等多种反应。目前，最常用的制备酰氯的方法是将羧酸与氯化试剂如 $SOCl_2$、三氯化磷、五氯化磷等反应。

氯化亚砜制备酰氯反应条件温和，在室温或稍加热即可反应。产物除酰氯外其他均为气体，往往不需提纯即可应用，纯度好，产率高。如果所生成酰氯的沸点与氯化亚砜的沸点相近，则酰氯与氯化亚砜不易分离。用三氯化磷制备酰氯时，适用于制备低沸点的酰氯，因反应中生成的亚磷酸不易挥发，可方便蒸出酰氯。五氯化磷适用于制备高沸点酰氯，以便于蒸出 $POCl_3$ 而得到酰氯。

在本实验中，丙酰氯采用丙酸与三氯化磷在 50℃反应 3 h 即可制得。

反应式：

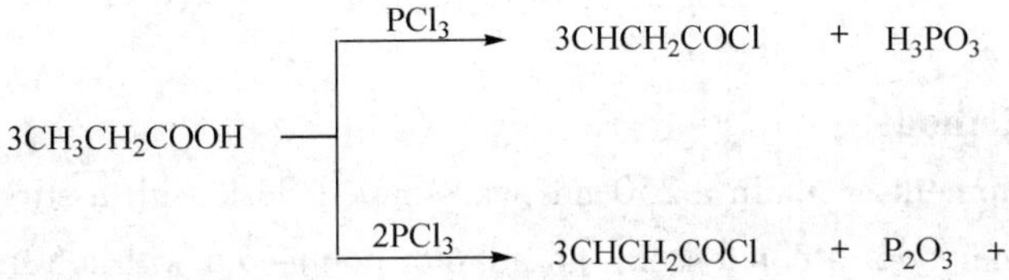

【实验方法】

在集热式磁力搅拌器的油浴锅中，安装具有搅拌子的 250ml 茄形瓶，茄形瓶口依次安装蒸馏头、温度计、直形冷凝管和尾接管。尾接管的两个支管分别连接一个 50ml 茄形瓶（用于收集前馏分）、一个 100ml 锥形瓶（用于收集产物，应预先称重）。尾接管还要用胶管依次连接氯化钙干燥管和气体吸收装置。

在茄形瓶中加入丙酸 18.5ml（0.25mol）和三氯化磷 8.7ml（0.1mol），升温至 50℃反应 3 h。反应毕，开始蒸馏，收集前馏分于 50ml 茄形瓶，收集主馏分于干燥并称重的 100ml 锥形瓶，具塞，称重，计算收率。

[**注释**] 1. 本实验为无水操作，三氯化磷和丙酰氯都会遇水分解。

2. 三氯化磷具有腐蚀性，称量时需要小心，不要与皮肤接触。

3. 蒸馏丙酰氯时，外浴温度不宜过高（低于 130℃），以避免亚磷酸焦化。

4. 本实验前馏分较少，待温度稳定后即可收集。未反应的三氯化磷与产品丙酰氯的沸点比较接近，通过蒸馏难以纯化产品。由于三氯化磷在苯丙酮的制备即傅－克（Fridel－Crafts）反应中没有不良影响，因此在收集丙酰氯时可带入少量三氯化磷。

5. 保存产品的锥形瓶瓶塞不要塞得过紧，且避免振摇，以防止分解气体冲出瓶塞造成危险。

6. 生成的亚磷酸粘于瓶底，且有强烈的刺激性。洗涤时可待茄形瓶稍冷后，加入适量的稀氢氧化钠溶液进行洗涤（需要在通风橱中完成）。

【思考题】

1. 除三氯化磷外，还可以用哪些试剂制备丙酰氯？各有何特点？

2. 三氯化磷与丙酸混合均匀放置片刻，溶液将为两分层。试解释此现象。

Ⅰ. Preparation of Propionyl chloride

Purpose

1. To master the preparation method for acyl chloride.

2. To master the distillation procedure.

Mechanism

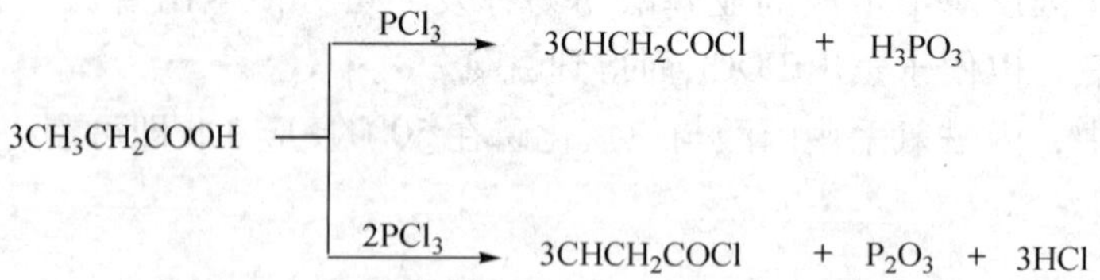

Experimental Methods

The reaction equipments contain a 250 ml pear-shaped flask with a stirring bar, a distilling head and a thermometer, a condenser, an adaptor connected with a 50ml flask (to collect the former fraction) and a 100 ml conical flask (it should be weighed beforehand) respectively. A drying tube containing calcium chloride and a gas absorption device should be connected with an the adaptor by a hose in sequence. A magnetic stirring apparatus with oil bath is used in the experiment.

18. 5 ml(0. 25 mol) of carboxylic acid and 8. 7 ml(0. 1 mol) of phosphorus trichloride are added into the flask and the reactants are heated to 50℃ for 3 h. Then the mixture is heated with an oil bath, the former fraction is collected to a 50 ml flask, and the main fraction is collected to the conical flask(it should be dried and weighed beforehand). A stopper is put on the conical flask and the yield is calculated[6].

Notes:

(1) Phosphorus trichloride and propionyl chloride should be decomposed when meeting water, therefore, the whole process should be water-free.

(2) Phosphorus trichloride is a strongly corrosive reagent! Be careful! And keep it away from your skin when weighing phosphorus trichloride.

(3) During the distillation of propionyl chloride, the temperature of oil bath should be less than 130℃ in order to prevent H_3PO_3 from coking.

(4) The main fraction is collected when the temperature is stable. The boiling points of phosphorus trichloride and propionyl chloride are close, therefore the distilled product propionyl chloride contains somewhat phosphorus trichloride. Phosphorus trichloride does not affect the following Fridel-Crafts reaction, therefore a little phosphorus trichloride remained in propionyl chloride is allowed.

(5) The conical flask with propionyl chloride should not be too tight and shaken to avoid the gas out of the flask.

(6) Phosphorous acid, a sticky liquid, had a strong irritating odor. The pear - shaped flask with phosphorous acid is cleaned with diluted NaOH solution when the flask is cold. This process should be carried out in the draught cupboard.

Questions

1. What other reagents could be used in the reaction besides phosphorus trichloride? And what are their differences?

2. The solution will be separated into two phases when phosphorus trichloride and propionic acid are mixed for a while. Try to explain this phenomenon.

二、苯丙酮的制备

【目的要求】

1. 掌握傅-克（Fridel-Crafts）反应的原理及基本操作。
2. 熟悉减压蒸馏的基本操作和注意事项。
3. 了解无水三氯化铝的性质、特点及使用时注意事项。

【实验原理】

合成路线如下：

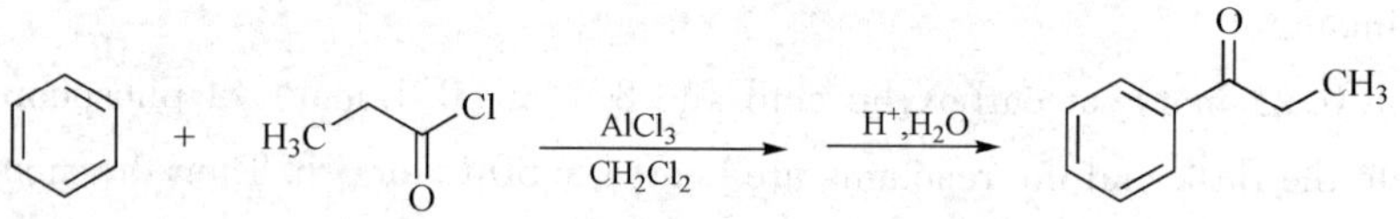

【实验方法】

（一）苯丙酮的制备

在集热式磁力搅拌器的水浴锅中，安装具有搅拌子的250 ml三颈瓶，三颈瓶口分别安装温度计、球形冷凝管和滴液漏斗。球形冷凝管上端安装氯化钙干燥管，后者再连接氯化氢气体吸收装置。

冰浴冷却下，将无水$AlCl_3$ 18.3 g（0.137 mol）、干燥的二氯甲烷30 ml加入至反应瓶中，搅拌，冰水浴冷却反应液至0℃～5℃。将丙酰氯11.7 g（0.126 mol）、苯7.6 ml（0.085 mol）、二氯甲烷20 ml混匀，置于滴液漏斗中向反应液中滴加，控制滴加速度使反应液温度低于10℃。加毕，移去冰浴，室温下反应2 h。反应毕，将反应液用冰水浴冷却至0℃～5℃，搅拌下，向反应液中滴入稀盐酸（盐酸5 ml以冰水50ml稀释），控制滴加速度使反应液温度低于10℃。滴加完毕后，室温下搅拌至固体物完全溶解，分出有机层。水层用二氯甲烷萃取（20 ml×2）。合并有机层，依次用等体积的水、5%氢氧化钠溶液、水洗涤。将有机层转移到250 ml锥形瓶中，无水硫酸钠干燥，得到苯丙酮的二氯甲烷溶液。

（二）苯丙酮的纯化

将苯丙酮的二氯甲烷溶液首先常压蒸去二氯甲烷，再稍微冷却，改为空气冷凝管，用油泵减压蒸出苯丙酮，收集92℃/11mmHg的馏分。称重，计算收率。

[**注释**] 1. 仪器必须充分干燥，否则影响反应顺利进行。

2. 无水三氯化铝的质量是实验成败的关键之一。称量、投料都要迅速，避免长时间暴露在空气中。

3. 开始时，有诱导期，滴加10滴左右温度升高。控制滴加速度。

4. 由于最终产物不多，宜选用较小的蒸馏瓶，二氯甲烷溶液可用滴液漏斗分次加入蒸馏瓶中。蒸完的二氯甲烷先回收，再减压蒸馏；减压时，打开油泵，先将缓冲瓶的旋塞缓缓关闭，将毛细管的夹子夹紧；完毕后，先将毛细管的夹子打开，再缓缓打开缓冲瓶的旋塞。

【思考题】

1. 水和潮气对本实验有何影响？在仪器装置和操作中应注意哪些事项？
2. 反应完成后，加入水或冰水或盐酸的目的是什么？
3. 在烷基化和酰基化反应中，无水三氯化铝的用量有何不同？为什么？

Ⅱ. Preparation of Propiophenone

Purposes

1. To master the mechanism and basic operation of Friedel-Crafts acylation reaction.

2. To grasp the procedure and notes of reduced pressure distillation.

3. To understand the properties, features and notes of anhydrous aluminium chloride.

Mechanism

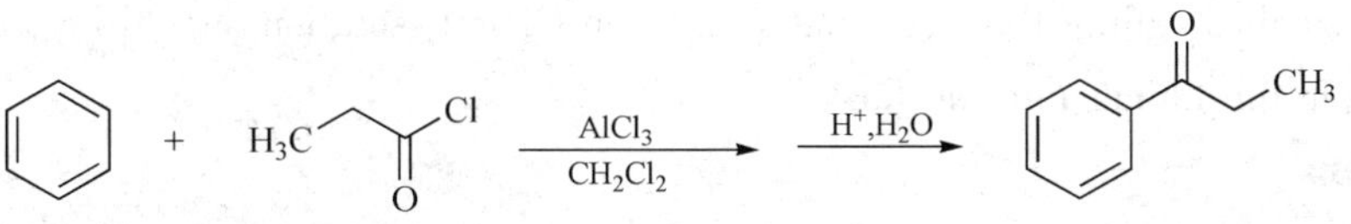

Experimental Methods

1. Preparation of Propiophenone

The reaction equipments contain a 250 ml three-necked flask with a stirring bar, a thermometer, a spherical condenser and a dropping funnel. A calcium chloride tube and a gas-absorbing device are connected on the top of the condenser. A magnetic stirring apparatus with a water bath is used in the experiment.

18.3 g (0.137mol) of finely powdered anhydrous aluminum chloride and 30 ml of anhydrous CH_2Cl_2 are added into a 250 ml three-necked flask. The mixture are stirred and cooled to 0-5℃ with an ice-water bath. Then 11.7 g(0.126 mol) of propionyl chloride, 7.6 ml(0.085 mol) of benzene and 20 ml of CH_2Cl_2 are added into the dropping funnel and the resultant mixture is added dropwise into the flask with ice-water cooling at such a rate that the internal temperature always remains below 10℃. After that, the temperature of the mixture is raised slowly to room temperature and is stirring for 2 h continuously.

The reaction mixture is cooled to 0-5℃ with an ice-water bath, and then diluted hydrochloride solution (5 ml in 50 ml cold water) is added dropwise into the flask under stirring at such a rate that the internal temperature always remains below 10℃. When the ketone-aluminum chloride complex is decomposed, the organic layer is separated off in the separating funnel and the aqueous layer is extracted with two 20 ml portions of CH_2Cl_2. The organic layers are combined together and carefully ished with water, 5% sodium hydroxide solution, water in sequence. The organic layer is transferred to a 250 ml conical flask and dried over anhydrous sodium sulfate, then the dichloromethane solution of propiophenone is obtained.

2. Purification of propiophenone

The solvent (CH_2Cl_2) is evaporated off firstly, then cooled slightly. Finally the propiophenone is distilled by an oil pump *in vacuum*, b. p 92℃/11mmHg. The product is weighed and the yield is calculated.

Notes:

(1) The equipments should be pre-dry well, otherwise it would affect the reaction.

(2) The success of the experiment depends on the quality of anhydrous aluminum chloride. The operation on anhydrous aluminum chloride should be quick to avoid its exposure to the air.

(3) There is an induction period in the reaction and the temperature is raised rapidly when about ten drops are added from the dropping funnel. The dropping speed should be controlled carefully.

(4) A small distilling flask is suitable and the CH_2Cl_2 solution should be added portion-by-portion from the funnel into the flask.

Questions

1. How do water and moisture affect the reaction and what issues should we pay attention to during the operation?

2. What is the purpose for the addition of water or hydrochloride after the completion of the reaction?

3. The amounts of anhydrous aluminum chloride are different in alkylation reaction and acylation reaction. Briefly state the reasons.

三、α-甲基-β-二甲氨基苯丙酮的制备

【目的要求】

1. 通过曼尼希（Mannich）反应制备α-甲基-β-二甲氨基苯丙酮盐酸盐，掌握曼尼希（Mannich）碱的制备方法。

2. 熟悉有机碱化合物的性质及纯化方法。

【实验原理】

合成路线如下：

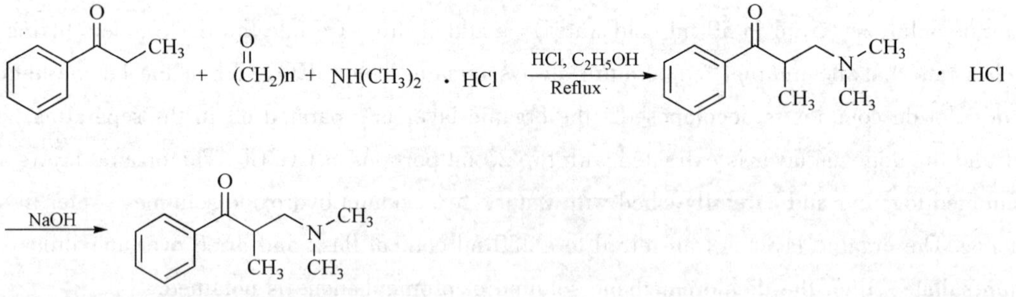

【实验方法】

（一）α-甲基-β-二甲氨基苯丙酮盐酸盐的制备

在250 ml锥形瓶中，加入苯丙酮13.4 g(0.1 mol)、多聚甲醛6.0 g(0.2 mol)、二甲胺盐酸盐8.2 g(0.1 mol)、乙醇75 ml和盐酸2 ml，加热回流5 h。反应毕，将反应

液转移至250 ml茄形瓶中，沸水浴加热，常压蒸馏大部分乙醇，稍降温后，用水泵减压蒸尽剩余的乙醇。冷却，有白色结晶析出，抽滤，滤饼用无水丙酮洗涤，干燥，得α-甲基-β-二甲氨基苯丙酮盐酸盐，称重，计算收率。

（二）α-甲基-β-二甲氨基苯丙酮乙醚溶液的制备

将α-甲基-β-二甲氨基苯丙酮盐酸盐置于烧杯中，加入20 ml水溶解。滴加20%氢氧化钠溶液至pH＞12。用乙醚萃取25ml×3，合并有机层，20ml水洗，转移至干燥的250 ml锥形瓶中，无水硫酸镁干燥，即得α-甲基-β-二甲氨基苯丙酮的乙醚溶液。

［**注释**］1. 加入盐酸2 ml回流1h后，若多聚甲醛没有全部解聚，可以补加盐酸1 ml，以促进其解聚；反应初期加热温度不要过高，回流的速度应缓慢，防止甲醛解聚过快而造成挥发。

2. 蒸馏乙醇时，用沸水浴为宜，可防止温度过高导致产物分解；α-甲基-β-二甲氨基苯丙酮盐酸盐易溶于水，因此应注意无水操作。

3. 无水丙酮洗涤α-甲基-β-二甲氨基苯丙酮盐酸盐的目的主要是除去未反应的苯丙酮。

4. α-甲基-β-二甲氨基苯丙酮盐酸盐干燥前的有机溶剂残留量约为50%。

【思考题】 Mannich反应在酸性条件下进行时，一般用胺类的盐酸盐，必要时加少量盐酸。酸的作用是什么？

Ⅲ. Preparation of α-methyl-β-dimethylaminophenylpropanone

Purposes

1. To master the synthetic method of the mannich bases by the preparation of α-methyl-β-dimethylaminophenylpropanone through Mannich reaction.

2. To know well the physico-chemical properties of organic bases and grasp their purification methods.

Mechanism

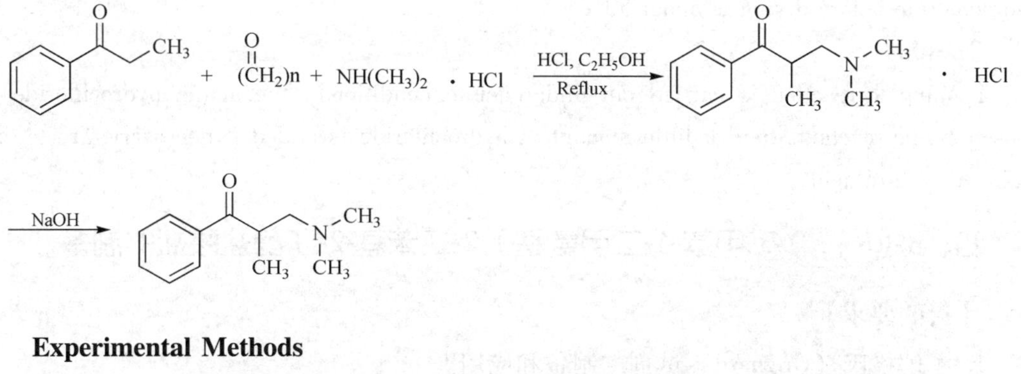

Experimental Methods

1. Preparation of α-methyl-β-dimethylaminophenylpropanone hydrochloride

13.4 g (0.1 mol) of propiophenone, 6.0 g (0.2 mol) of paraformaldehyde, 8.2 g

(0.1 mol) of dimethylamine hydrochloride in 75.0 ml of ethanol, with the addition of 2.0 ml of concentrate hydrochloric acid(to depolymerize the paraformaldehyde), are boiling in a 250 ml conical flask with a reflux condenser. After 5 h, the hot reaction mixture is transferred to a 250ml pear-shaped flask and heated in a boiling water bath, then most ethanol is evaporated off. The bath temperature is cooled to about 60℃, then the residual alcohol is removed through distillation in the vacuum of a water pump. The residue is cooled to room temperature, then white crystals precipitate. The hydrochloride of the Mannich base is filtered off and the filter cake is ished with a little amount of dry acetone. The product is dried in vacuum to constant weight. It is weighed and the yield is calculated.

2. Preparation of α-methyl-β-dimethylamino-phenylpropanone in ether solution

The Mannich base hydrochloride is placed into a beaker and 20ml of water is added to dissolve it. The pH of the solution is adjusted to higher than 12 with 20% sodium hydroxide solution. The mixture is extracted with three 25ml portions of ether, then the organic layers are combined and ished with 20 ml of water. The organic phase is transferred to a 250 ml conical flask, dried over magnesium sulfate, then the ether solution of α-methyl-β-dimethyllamino-phenylpropanone is obtained.

Notes:

(1) If there still exists undepolymerized paraformaldehyde after refluxing for 1 h, another 1.0 ml of concentrate hydrochloric acid should be added to promote depolymerization; the initial reaction temperature should not be too high to prevent the volatilization of the depolymerized formaldehyde.

(2) Boling water bath is chosen for the distillation of the alcohol to prevent the decomposition of the product due to the high temperature; Water-free! The product is highly hydroscopic, and easily soluble in water.

(3) The purpose of using anhydrous acetone to ish the product is to remove the unreacted propiophenone.

(4) The amount of residual solvent in 1-dimethylamino-2-methyl-3-phenylpropan-3-one hydrochloride before drying is about 50%.

Questions

1. Mannich reaction is carried out under acidic conditions, the amine hydrochloride is chosen as the reactant, and a little amount of hydrochloride is added if necessary. Try to explain the role of acid.

四、α-(*d*, *l*)-3-甲基-4-二甲氨基-1,2-二苯基-2-丁醇盐酸盐的制备

【目的要求】

1. 了解格氏（Grignard）试剂的制备和应用。
2. 掌握格氏（Grignard）试剂与酮反应制备叔醇的原理及操作。
3. 熟悉有机胺类化合物成盐酸盐的方法。

4. 掌握重结晶原理及常规操作方法。

【实验原理】

合成路线如下：

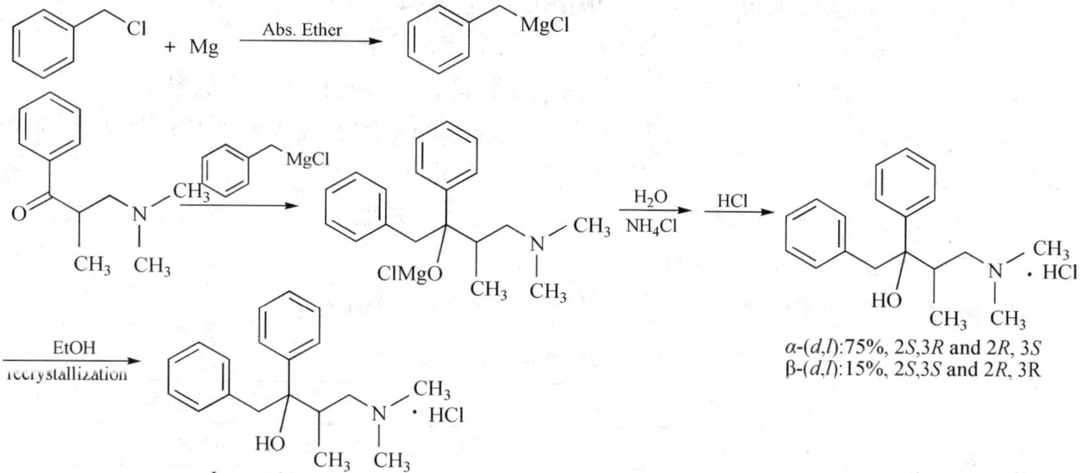

I　α-(*d,l*)

【实验方法】

（一）格氏（Grignard）试剂的制备

在集热式磁力搅拌器的水浴锅中，安装具有搅拌子的250ml三颈瓶，三颈瓶口分别安装温度计、球形冷凝管和滴液漏斗，球形冷凝管上端装一氯化钙干燥管。

在三颈瓶上中加入干燥镁屑1.5 g(0.0625 mol)、绝对乙醚、碘粒少许，在滴液漏斗中加入氯化苄7.2 ml(7.9 g，0.0625mol)；绝对乙醚的用量没过镁屑即可。先向三颈瓶中加入2~3ml氯化苄，当镁屑表面有气泡产生，反应液呈现混浊时即表明反应引发，开动搅拌，同时将滴液漏斗中其余的氯化苄加入等体积的绝对乙醚混合均匀，缓慢滴加，控制滴加速度以维持溶液呈微沸状态。滴加完毕，加热回流15~20 min，冷至室温，备用。

（二）4-二甲氨基-1,2-二苯基-3-甲基-2-丁醇的制备

将*α*-甲基-*β*-二甲氨基苯丙酮的乙醚溶液〔相当于其盐酸盐11.4 g（0.05 mol）〕在搅拌下滴入上述制备的苄基氯化镁乙醚溶液中，控制滴加速度维持反应液呈微沸状态。滴加完毕，继续加热回流2 h。反应毕，将反应液冷却至0℃~5℃，向反应液中缓慢滴加饱和氯化铵水溶液分解加成产物。分解完全后，将反应液移至分液漏斗中，分出有机层，水层用乙醚萃取15 ml ×2，合并乙醚层，等体积水洗涤，移至250 ml锥形瓶中，无水硫酸钠干燥，即得4-二甲氨基-1,2-二苯基-3-甲基-2-丁醇的乙醚溶液。

（三）4-二甲氨基-1,2-二苯基-3-甲基-2-丁醇盐酸盐的制备

将干燥后的4-二甲氨基-1,2-二苯基-3-甲基-2-丁醇的乙醚溶液移至干燥的250 ml三颈瓶中，搅拌下，向乙醚溶液中滴入氯化氢无水乙醇溶液直至无沉淀生成，抽滤，少量无水乙醇洗涤，干燥，得4-二甲氨基-1,2-二苯基-3-甲基-2-丁醇盐酸盐粗品〔其中，*α*-(*d*, *l*)：85%~90%，*β*-(*d*, *l*)：10%~15%〕，称重，计算收率。

(四) α-(*d*, *l*)-4-二甲氨基-1，2-二苯基-3-甲基-2-丁醇盐酸盐的制备

用甲醇－乙酸乙酯（4∶1）进行重结晶，得 α-(*d*, *l*)4-二甲氨基-1,2-二苯基-3-甲基-2-丁醇盐酸盐精品，干燥，称重，计算收率。

[**注释**] 1. 仪器必须充分干燥，否则影响反应顺利进行。

2. 镁屑使用前应在 60℃下干燥 4 h 以上，并且剪成小段。

3. 乙醚应绝对无水，严格纯化。其沸点比较低，应注意控制加热的温度。

4. 为了促进反应易于发生，应使开始时氯化苄局部浓度较大，而且所加入的碘粒要在氯化苄局部浓度最大处，搅拌应在反应开始后进行。

5. 氯化苄有着较强的刺激性，使用时不要接触到皮肤、眼睛，特别要小心氯化苄与乙醚的混合蒸汽对眼睛的接触。

6. 氯化铵的用量为，格氏试剂∶氯化铵＝1∶4（摩尔比）。

氯化铵溶解度

温度℃	0	10	20	30	40	50	60	70	80	90	100
溶解度	29.4	33.3	37.2	41.4	45.8	50.4	55.2	60.2	65.6	71.3	77.3

7. 氯化氢无水乙醇溶液的制备

装置：

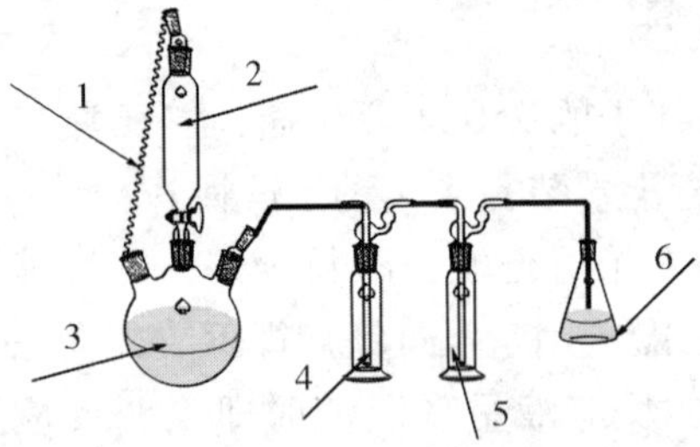

1. 恒压管
2. 100ml 滴液漏斗（硫酸 50ml）
3. 250ml 三颈瓶（50ml 盐酸）
4. 干燥瓶（硫酸适量）
5. 安全瓶
6. 100ml 锥形瓶（50ml 无水乙醇，冰水浴冷却）

方法：在 250ml 三颈瓶中加入盐酸 50ml；100ml 滴液漏斗中加入硫酸 50ml；洗气瓶中加入硫酸适量，以高于洗气管内细管 2～3mm 为宜；100ml 锥形瓶加入无水乙醇 50ml。将硫酸缓慢滴入盐酸中，则生成的氯化氢通过洗气瓶的干燥，注入用冰水浴冷却的无水乙醇中，得氯化氢无水乙醇溶液。

8. α 型产物在甲醇－乙酸乙酯（4∶1）中的溶解度低于 β 型，因此通过重结晶除去少量的 β 型产物。

【思考题】 1. 本实验在将格氏（Grignard）试剂加成物水解前的各步中，为什么使用的药品和仪器必须绝对干燥？为此应采取什么措施？

2. 为什么用乙醚作为格氏（Grignard）反应的溶剂？还可以选用什么做溶剂？

3. 氯苄滴加太快或一次加入，有什么不好？

4. 本实验中为什么用饱和氯化铵溶液水解加成产物，而不是用盐酸？

5. 通常状态下空气中的水分用无水氯化钙干燥，氯化氢用浓硫酸干燥，那么氨气用什么干燥呢？

6. 写出 *α*-甲基-*β*-二甲氨基苯丙酮与苄基氯化镁反应产物的旋光异构体，并指出优势产物，并解释原因。

Ⅳ. Preparation of 4-dimethylamino-1,2-diphenyl-3-methyl-2-butanol hydrochloride

Purposes

1. To grasp the preparation method of Grignard reagents as well as their applications
2. To grasp the principle and relative manipulation for the preparation of tertiary alcohols through the reaction of Grignard reagents with ketones.
3. To understand the preparation method of organic amine hydrochlorides
4. To master the principle and process of recrystallization.

Mechanism

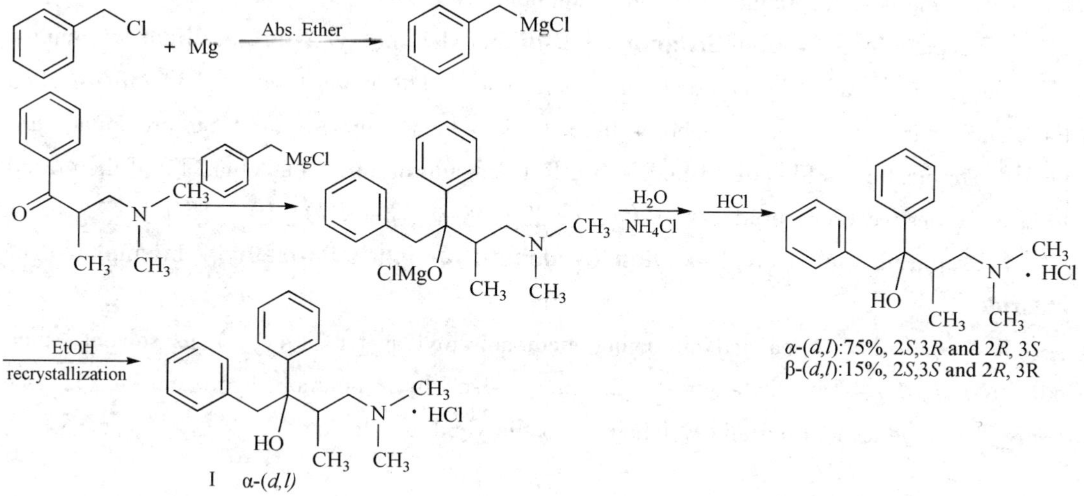

I α-(*d,l*)

Experimental methods

1. preparation of Grignard reagent:

The reaction equipments contain a 250 ml three-necked flask with a dropping funnel, a stirring bar, a reflux condenser with an anhydrous calcium chloride tube on the top and a thermometer. A magnetic stirring apparatus with a water bath is used in the experiment.

1.5 g(0.0625 mol) of pre-dried magnesium turnings, absolute anhydrous ether and a few grains of iodine are added into the three-necked flask, and 7.2 ml(7.9 g, 0.0625mol) of benzyl chloride is added from the dropping funnel. 2-3 ml of benzyl chloride is dropped into the flask first and then bubbles appear on the surface of magnesium turnings and the reaction solution becomes cloudy which shows the start of the reaction (If the reaction doesn't start, 0.5 ml of bromine or a few drops of carbon tetrachloride are added to the reaction mixture, which is gently heated). The reaction mixture is stirred after the reaction started. Meanwhile, the remaining benzyl chloride, which is dissolved in the same volume of absolute ether, is added dropwise with further stirring in such a way that the ether boiled gently. After the addition, the mixture is boiled gently on the water bath until almost all the magnesium is dissolved (about 15-20 min) and then the mixture is cooled to ambient temperature for the use of next step.

2. Preparation of 4-dimethylamino-1,2-diphenyl-3-methyl-2-butanol

The mannich base ethereal solution (equivalent to its hydrochloride 11.4 g, 0.05mol) is added dropwise into the solution of the Grignard reagent (the adding speed should be well - controlled to make the solution in the state of slightly boiling). After the addition is completed, the mixture is heated on the water bath with stirring for another 2 hours, and then the solution is cooled by an ice bath. The saturated aqueous ammonium chloride[6] is added to the previous solution to hydrolyze the additive product. The ethereal layer is separated off and the aqueous phase is extracted twice with ether, 15 ml for each time. The combined extracts are ished with water of same volume and then transferred to a 250 ml conical flask and dried over sodium sulfate to give the desired product's ethereal solution.

3. Preparation of 4-dimethylamino-1,2-diphenyl-3-methyl-2-butanol hydrochloride:

The desired product's ethereal solution is placed into a pre-dried 250 ml three-necked flask and hydrogen chloride alcohol solution[7] is added dropwise until no precipitate appeared. The mixture is filtered, ished with a little amount of anhydrous ethanol and then dried to give the desired crude product [α-(*d*,*l*): 85%-90%, β-(*d*,*l*): 10%-15%].

4. Preparation of α-(*d*,*l*)-4-Dimethylamino-1,2-diphenyl-3-methyl-2-butanol hydrochloride

Recrystallization is carried out using methanol-ethyl acetate (4 : 1) as solvent, then pure α-(*d*, *l*)-4-Dimethylamino-1, 2-diphenyl-3-methyl-2-butanol hydrochloride is obtained. The product is dried and weighed, and the yield is calculated.

Notes:

(1) The apparatus should be intensively dried to avoid affecting the reaction.

(2) The magnesium turning should be dried for more than 4 h at 60℃ and cut into chips before use.

(3) Ether should be absolutely anhydrous with high purity. Since its boiling point is relatively low, the reaction temperature should be strictly controlled.

(4) The initial local concentration of benzyl chloride should be high, and the iodine granule should be added in the place with high concentration of benzyl chloride. The reaction mixture should not be stirred until the reaction begins.

(5) Benzyl chloride possesses high irritability and it should be prevented from skin and eyes.

(6) The amount of ammonium chloride is 4 folders as that of Grignard reagent (mole ratio).

Solubility of ammonium chloride in water

Temperature (℃)	0	10	20	30	40	50	60	70	80	90	100
Solubility (g)	29.4	33.3	37.2	41.4	45.8	50.4	55.2	60.2	65.6	71.3	77.3

7. Preparation of hydrogen chloride ethyl alcohol solution

Equipments:

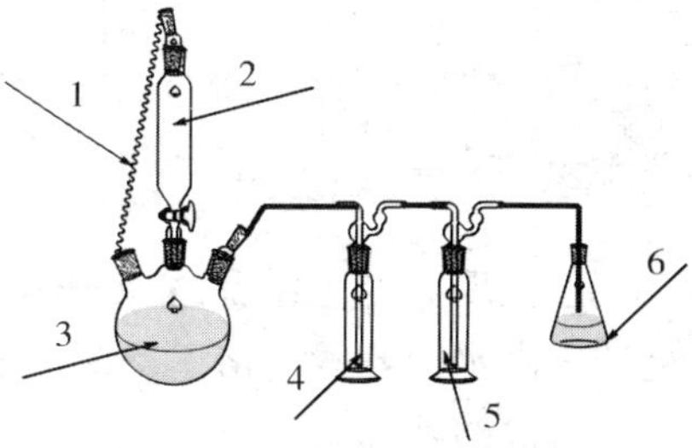

1. pipe for constant pressure

2. 100 ml dropping funnel containing 50 ml of sulfuric acid

3. 250 ml three – necked flask containing 50 ml of hydrochloric acid

4. dry flask containing suitable amount of sulfuric acid)

5. safety bottle

6. 100 ml conical flask containing 50 ml anhydrous alcohol, cooled by an ice bath.

Procedure: 50 ml of hydrochloric acid is added into a 250 ml three-necked flask. 50 ml sulfuric acid is added into a 100 ml dropping funnel. Suitable sulfuric acid is added into the gas ishing bottle. 50 ml of anhydrous alcohol is placed into a 100 ml conical flask. Sulfuric acid is added dropwise from the funnel into the hydrochloric acid, and then the hydrogen chloride gas gets out, which is dried through the gas ishing bottle and finally absorbed by the anhydrous alcohol cooled in ice bath. Then the hydrogen chloride alcohol solution is obtained.

8. The mixture is separated into α and β components by crystallization from methanol – ethyl acetate, the diastereoisomer α being the less soluble component.

Questions

1. Try to explain the reason that all the apparatuses and reagents should be absolutely dried before the hydrolysis step. What measures should be taken ?

2. We use ether as the solvent for the Grignard reaction, what else can be used?

3. What are the problems if we add benzyl chloride quickly or add it in one – portion?

4. Why use saturated ammonium chloride other than hydrochloric acid to hydrolyze the addition product?

5. Generally, water in the air can be dried using calcium chloride; hydrogen chloride can be dried by concentrated sulfuric acid. What can be used for ammonia gas?

6. Write the structures of each stereoisomer, and state the predominant isomer and explain the reason.

实验二十六　巴比妥（Barbitone）的合成

【目的要求】

1. 通过巴比妥的合成了解药物合成的基本过程。

2. 掌握无水操作技术。

【实验原理】

巴比妥（Barbitone），化学名为5,5-二乙基-2,4,6-(1*H*,3*H*,5*H*)嘧啶三酮。巴比妥为长效镇静催眠药，具镇静、催眠、抗惊厥及抗癫痫作用。还可用作麻醉前给药，与解热镇痛药合用时可增强后者的镇痛作用。

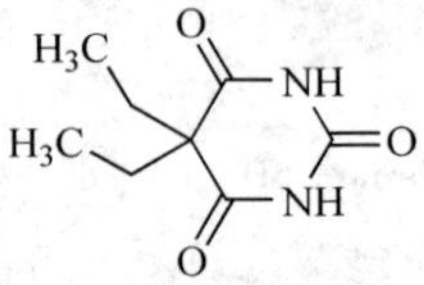

巴比妥为白色结晶或结晶性粉末，无臭，味微苦。mp. 189℃ ~192℃。难溶于水，易溶于沸水及乙醇，溶于乙醚、三氯甲烷及丙酮。

合成路线如下：

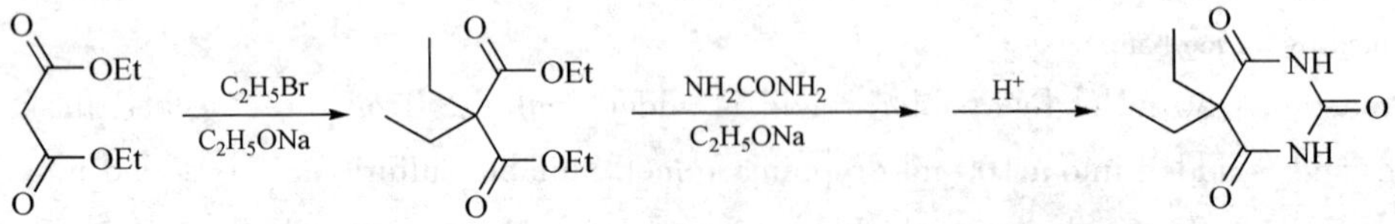

Experiment 26 Synthesis of Barbitone

Purpose

1. To understand the basic process of drug synthesis through the synthesis of Barbital.
2. To grasp the anhydrous operation.

Mechanism

Barbitone (5,5-diethylbarbituric acid), 5,5-diethylpyrimidine-2,4,6-(1*H*,3*H*,5*H*)-trione, is a long-acting sedative-hypnotic with sedative, hypnotic, anticonvulsant and antiepileptic effects. It can also be used as preanesthetic medication, and enhance analgesic effect of antipyretic analgesics in combination with the latter.

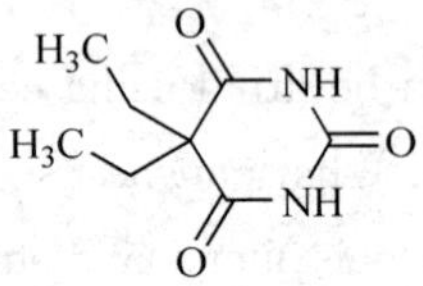

Barbital is an odorless and faintly bitter white crystal or crystal powder, mp. 189-192℃, insoluble in the water, but solve in boiling water and ethanol easily, soluble in diethyl ether, chloroform and acetone.

Synthetic route is as follows:

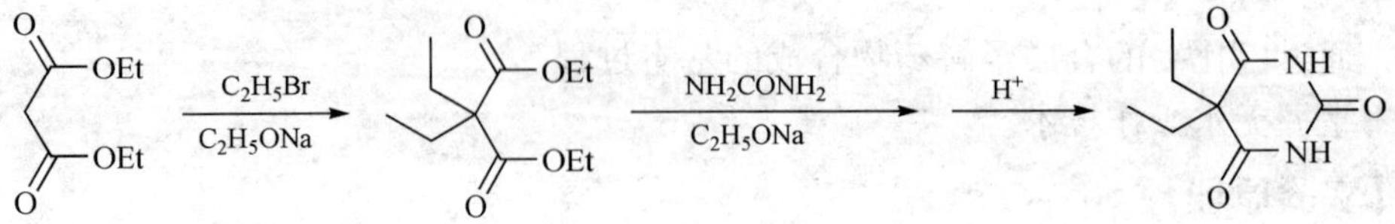

一、二乙基丙二酸二乙酯的制备

【目的要求】

学习丙二酸二乙酯烃化反应的原理和方法。

【实验原理】

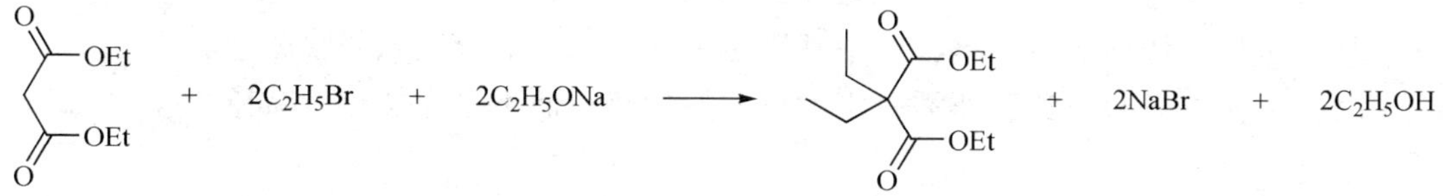

【实验方法】

在集热式磁力搅拌器的油浴锅中，安装内置有搅拌子的250ml三颈瓶，在三颈瓶的三口上分别安装具有无水氯化钙干燥管的球形冷凝管、温度计和空心塞。向三颈瓶中依次加入无水乙醇29 ml和金属钠丝2.3 g(0.1 mol)。油浴加热使无水乙醇回流并搅拌（油浴温度不超过90℃），直至金属钠丝全部溶解。冷却反应液至有少量乙醇钠晶体析出，加入5滴乙酸乙酯，继续搅拌10 min。室温下向乙醇钠溶液中加入丙二酸二乙酯7.5 ml（0.05 mol），搅拌15 min后，油浴加热回流30 min。此时固体全部溶解。再次冷却，即有少量丙二酸二乙酯二钠晶体析出。将丙二酸二乙酯二钠的乙醇溶液降温到30℃以下，向反应液加入溴乙烷7.5 ml(0.1 mol)，在30℃~35℃下搅拌30 min，之后以2℃/min的速度缓慢升温直至回流，然后再回流2 h。反应毕，将反应液冷却至室温。将球形冷凝管改为常压蒸馏头，并且依次连接直形冷凝管、双支真空接收管和茄形瓶。搅拌并缓缓加热，逐滴蒸出乙醇。直至每分钟仅有5滴乙醇蒸出时，将反应物和油浴的温度都降到30℃~40℃，将已蒸出的乙醇回收，然后用水循环真空泵减压蒸除残余乙醇，直到反应物50℃（不得高于这个温度!）于真空状态下不再有乙醇被蒸出。冷却反应物至室温，加水适量使反应物中的固体溶解。转移至分液漏斗中，分出有机层，水层用乙醚萃取10ml×4次，合并有机层，20ml水洗，将有机层转移至100ml锥形瓶中，无水硫酸钠干燥，具塞，放置。

安装减压蒸馏装置，将干燥后的二乙基丙二酸二乙酯乙醚萃取液滤去干燥剂，加入减压蒸馏瓶中，电热套加热，常压蒸尽乙醚。减压蒸馏，收集82~85℃/11mmHg馏分，保存在干燥并称重的100ml锥形瓶中，具塞，称重，计算收率。

［**注释**］1. 本实验为无水反应，所用的反应仪器、量具及试剂必须充分干燥。

2. 金属钠与乙醇的反应是放热反应，加入金属钠丝之前，无水乙醇不得加热，避免爆沸。

3. 减压蒸馏装置的各个仪器相互连接处，必须清洁并涂有凡士林。

【思考题】

1. 使用金属钠时应注意哪些事项？

2. 为什么要向已经制备好的乙醇钠溶液中加入少许乙酸乙酯？

3. 为什么在加入溴乙烷之前，必须将反应液降至30℃以下。

4. 在二乙基丙二酸二乙酯的制备中，用水循环真空泵减压蒸馏乙醇时，为什么在真空状态下一定要控制反应物温度不得高于50℃？

5. 在二乙基丙二酸二乙酯的制备中，“冷却反应物至室温，加水适量使反应物中的固体溶解”。这里所述的“固体”是什么？为什么要加水溶解？

6. 在减压蒸馏时，为什么必须遵守如下操作，否则如何？

（1）减压蒸馏前，应将接收瓶中常压蒸出的低沸点馏分倒入回收瓶中。

（2）一定要先减压达到所需真空度后开始加热；而不是先加热后减压。

Ⅰ. Synthesis of Diethyl diethylmalonate

Purpose

To master the principle and the method of alkylation of diethyl malonate

Mechanism

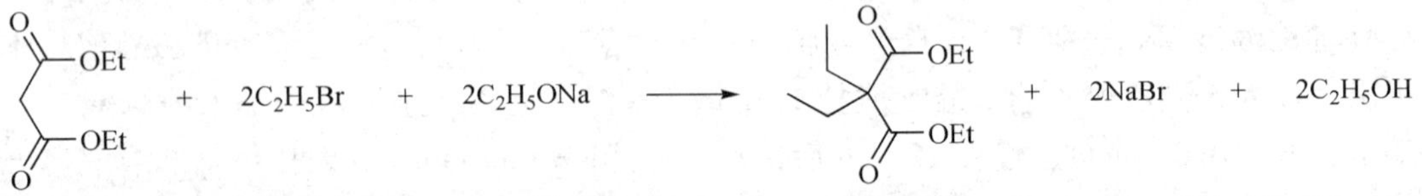

Experimental methods

The reaction equipments contain a 250ml three-necked flask with a stirring bar, a spherical condenser (with a dry tube containing calcium chloride), a thermometer and a stopper. 2. 3g (0. 1mol) of clean sodium is placed in the flask and 29 ml of anhydrous ethanol is added. The resultant mixture is stirred and warmed to reflux on an oil bath (the temperature of the oil bath should not be higher than 90℃) in order to complete the solution of the sodium. The sodium ethoxide solution is cooled and 5 drops of ethyl acetate are added when the sodium ethoxide commences to separate out. Then the reaction mixture is kept stirring for another 10 mins. 7. 5 ml (0. 05mol) of ethyl malonate (dried over anhydrous calcium sulfate) is added to the above solution at ambient temperature and keep stirring for 15 mins. The mixture is refluxed for 30 mins on an oil bath to dissolve the solid. When the mixture is cooled to below 30℃ (the ethyl sodium malonate commences to crystallize out), 7. 5 ml (0. 1mol) of dry ethyl bromide is added. The reaction mixture is stirred at 30 – 35℃ for 30 mins and then raised to reflux temperature at the speed of 2℃/min, and kept refluxing for 2 h to complete the reaction. Then the reaction mixture is cooled to the ambient temperature. The equipment for distillation is rearranged and alcohol is distilled off as much as possible on an oil bath. It is advisable to get off the remaining alcohol, attention! The temperature of the oil bath should be less than 50℃. The mixture is cooled to ambient temperature, then diluted with water to dissolve the solid, then transferred to a separating funnel. The organic layer is separated off and aqueous layer is extracted with ether (four 10 ml portions) . The combined ether is ished with 20 ml of water, transferred to a 100 ml conical flask, dried with anhydrous sodium sulfate and closed with a stopper.

After the drying agent filtered off, the etheris removed on an electric jacket, then the residue is distilled *in vacuum*. The ethyl diethylmalonate is collected at 82 – 85℃/11mmHg and transferred to a 100ml conical flask (it should be dried and weighed beforehand) with a stopper. The product is weighed and the yield is calculated.

Notes:

(1) It is important that the apparatus and reagents should be perfectly dry

(2) It is an exothermal reaction when sodium meets with alcohol. The alcohol should not be warmed before sodium is added!

(3) Each juncture part of the vacuum distillation apparatus should be cleaned and smeared with vaseline.

Questions

1. What items need your attention when use sodium?

2. Why add a little amount of ethyl acetate to the prepared sodium ethoxide solution?

3. The temperature of the reaction mixture should be cooled to less than 30℃ before the addition of ethyl bromide, try to explain the reason.

4. When prepare diethyl diethylmalonate, we use vacuum distillation to get off the alcohol residue, the temperature of the oil bath should be less than 50℃, try to explain the reason.

5. When preparing diethyl diethylmalonate, we cool the mixture and dilute the solid in the flask with water, what is the solid? Why use water to dissolve it?

6. What are the problems if we do not comply with the following operation when performing vacuum distillation?

(1) The low-boiling fraction in the receiving flask should be transferred to the recycling flask before vacuum distillation.

(2) Heating is not allowed until the desired vacuum pressure level is reached.

二、巴比妥的制备

【目的要求】

1. 掌握巴比妥类药物的一般合成方法。

2. 熟悉重结晶的操作。

【实验原理】

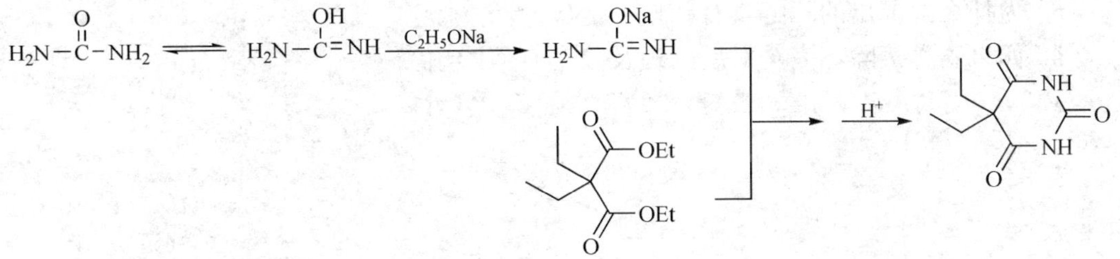

【实验方法】

（一）巴比妥的制备

在集热式磁力搅拌器的油浴锅中，在内置有搅拌子的250 ml烧瓶内加入金属钠1.7g(0.075mol)，然后迅速安装具有无水氯化钙干燥管的球形冷凝管。量取无水乙醇44 ml(0.75mol) 从球形冷凝管的上口一次性加入烧瓶中，搅拌。待回流较慢时，升温回流，直至金属钠丝反应完全。将反应液稍冷至有少量乙醇钠晶体析出时，滴入乙酸乙酯5滴，继续搅拌10 min。

向上述乙醇钠溶液中加入二乙基丙二酸二乙酯6.5 g(0.03mol) 和无水尿素2.3 g (0.0375mol)，加热使反应液呈微沸状态1.5 h。反应毕，将球形冷凝管改为常压蒸馏头，并且依次连接直形冷凝管、双支真空接收管和茄形瓶。搅拌并缓缓加热，以10～15滴/min的速度蒸出乙醇，直至外浴升温至110℃～115℃且不再有乙醇被蒸出（约需1.5 h）。将已蒸出的乙醇回收，用水循环真空泵减压蒸尽残余乙醇。

冷却反应物到室温后，向烧瓶内加入适量水使反应物溶解，若有不溶物应过滤除去。将此溶液转移至烧杯中，滴加15%硫酸溶液，调至pH 3～4，析出大量固体，抽滤，滤饼水洗至中性，干燥，得到巴比妥粗品，称重，计算收率。

（二）巴比妥的精制

安装回流装置，在烧瓶内放入巴比妥粗品，按照比例（巴比妥：水=1g：13ml）加入水，加热使其全部溶解。稍冷后加入适量活性炭（巴比妥粗品重量的1%～5%），继续加热微沸5～10 min，趁热过滤，将滤液缓慢冷却至室温，待结晶完全后抽滤，水洗，得巴比妥精品，干燥，称重，计算收率。

[**注释**] 1. 本缩合反应实验要求无水操作，否则影响收率，甚至完全失败。

2. 金属钠与乙醇的反应是放热反应，应适时加热，避免暴沸。

3. 在巴比妥钠的制备时，控制温度不宜过高，否则易使产物焦化。

4. 随着乙醇的蒸出，反应瓶内将逐渐有固体析出。固体的存在影响液体的热传递，这样可能会发生暴沸。为了避免暴沸，升温速度宜慢，搅拌速度宜匀。

4. 一定要将反应物冷却至室温后，才可以加水使之溶解，以防止生成的巴比妥钠在温度较高时发生酰胺键的断裂。

【思考题】

1. 在乙醇钠的制备方法上，本次实验与上次实验（二乙基丙二酸二乙酯的制备）比较，乙醇和钠的加料顺序完全相反。请分析各有何优缺点？

2. 本实验用水循环真空泵减压蒸馏乙醇时，为什么不像上次实验（二乙基丙二酸二乙酯的制备）时，要特别强调在真空状态下一定要控制反应物温度不得高于50℃？

3. 为什么蒸馏出的乙醇具有碱性？

4. 如果乙醇蒸除不完全对后处理及收率有何影响？

Ⅱ. Synthesis of Barbitone

Purposes

1. To master the preparation method of barbituric acid and its derivatives
2. To grasp the procedure of recrystallization.

Mechanism

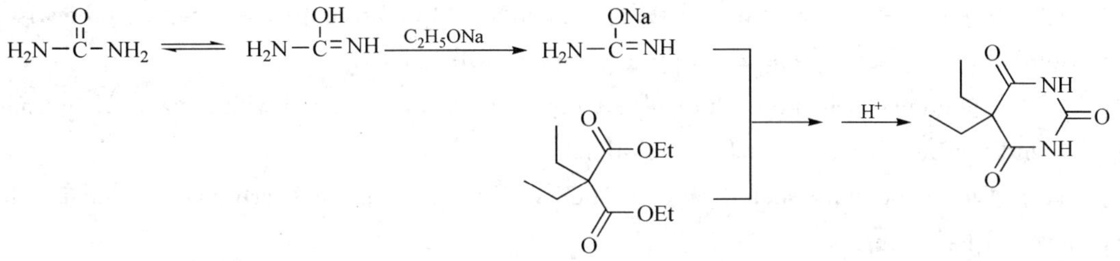

Experimental methods

1. Preparation ofbarbitone

The reaction equipments contain a 250ml flask with a stirring bar, a spherical condenser connected with a $CaCl_2$ dry tube. The magnetic stirring apparatus with an oil bath is used in the experiment. 1. 7g(0. 075mol) of clean sodium is placed in the flask and the reflux condenser with a $CaCl_2$ dry tube is fitted quickly. 44 ml (0. 75mol) of anhydrous ethanol is added and the resultant mixture is kept refluxing and stirring until all the sodium reacted. The reactants are cooled and some sodium ethoxide precipitates. Then 5 drops of ethyl acetate are added to the reactants and keep stirring for 10 min.

6. 5 g(0. 03mol) of diethyl diethylmalonate and 2. 3 g(0. 0375mol) of dry urea are added to the flask and the reactants are stirred and heated to boil gentlely for 1. 5h. When the reaction is finished, the equipment is changed to distillation equipment. Ethanol is slowly distilled off with the speed of 10-15 drops/min by the adjustment of temperature of the oil bath. When no ethanol appears (at least 1. 5 hr is needed for this procedure), the temperature should be increased to 110-115℃. Then vacuum distillation is performed until no ethanol appears under vacuum. Recycle ethanol and cooled the residue to ambient temperature. A suitable amount of water is added until the solid(sodium barbital) is dissolved (If some insoluble matter still existed, it should be filtered out). The solution is poured into a beaker and adjusted to pH 3-4 with 15% sulfuric acid. Barbitone is crystallized out when sufficient acid is used. The solids are filtered, ished with water to neutral and dried to give the crude barbitone. The product is weighed and the yield is calculated.

2. Refinement ofbarbitone

The crude barbitone and a suitable amount of water (13ml/g) are added into the beaker and the mixture is heated with stirring until all the barbital dissolved at the boiling point. Then the solution is cooled for a while and a suitable amount of activated carbon (1%-5% amount of the crude barbital) is added. The resultant mixture is heated and stirred again to slightly boil for 5-10 min (If the water is evaporated out, add a suitable amount of water), then filtered while hot. The hot filtrate is slowly cooled to room temperature, and the crystals are filtered off and dried in the air. The product is weighed and the yields (including recrystallization and the overall yield for the whole procedure starting from diethylmalonate) are calculated.

Notes:

(1) The equipments and the whole operation should be absolutely water-free; otherwise, the yield will be affected, and even the experiment will fail.

(2) Attention: It is an exothermal reaction when sodium reacted with alcohol. Heat timely to avoid the bursting boiling of the solution.

(3) The temperature should be controlled well when preparing barbitone, otherwise the product will be coking.

(4) The solid is precipitated out gradually as the alcohol is distilled out, which will affect the thermal transmission and cause the burst boiling of the solution. Therefore, the mixture temperature should be raised gradually with well stirring.

(5) Water should not be added to sodium barbiturate until the salt is cooled to room temperature in order to avoid the decomposition of the amide under high temperature.

Questions

1. When preparing sodium ethoxide, the charging sequence of ethanol and sodium in this experiment is quite different from that in last step (synthesis of diethyl diethylmalonate), try to explain the reason.

2. In the last step (synthesis of diethyl diethylmalonate), the temperature in vacuum distillation should be less than 50℃, however, no temperature limit is mentioned in this experiment, try to explain the reason.

3. The distillated alcohol is alkaline, try to explain the reason.

4. How will it affect the aftertreatment and yield if ethanol is not distilled out completely?

实验二十七　药物化学开放设计实验

一、肾上腺素β受体阻断剂的设计与合成

【实验目的】

1. 学生独立设计一个肾上腺素β受体阻断剂，并设计一条合理的合成路线，完成目标化合物的合成及鉴定工作。

2. 培养学生的药化实验技能及分析解决问题的能力，使学生在规定的（64 学时）实验时间内，独立完成实验内容，使学生初步体会科研的内涵与魅力。

3. 培养学生的团队协作精神。

【实验原理】

以现有的肾上腺素 β 受体阻断剂的构效关系及现有药物为基础，合理设计一个新的肾上腺素 β 受体阻断剂，并设计一条可行的合成路线，完成目标化合物的合成及鉴定。

【仪器设备】

电动搅拌机、电磁搅拌机、旋转蒸发仪（附有低温液体循环仪）、低温浴槽（-30℃）、高压釜、紫外检测器、高效液相和常规玻璃仪器。

【实验方式】

全天候开放式。

【实验学时】

64 学时。

【实验内容】

归纳总结现有的肾上腺素 β 受体阻断剂的构效关系。并根据肾上腺素 β 受体阻断剂的构效关系，自行设计一个结构全新的肾上腺素 β 受体阻断剂。根据设计的目标化合物结构，通过 CAS Scifinder 数据库及 Tomson integrity 数据库检索目标化合物的合成路线，并从学校现有的 Elsevier、CAS、CNKI 及中国知网等数据库资源下载原始文献，参考同类药物的合成路线，设计目标化合物的合成路线，一般以不超过六步反应为佳，并初步确定每步操作的实验条件。

实验开始 4 周前，要提交可行性实验报告，并与指导教师探讨目标化合物的合理性及设计路线的可行性。确定一条合理可行的合成路线，提交实验内容需要的化学原料、试剂及仪器清单。由实验中心完成前期准备工作。

学生以 3 ~4 人组成实验组，在规定时间内（一般 64 学时）独立完成实验内容。实验过程中，学生应通过薄层紫外鉴定等常规分析手段判断各步反应中间体及目标产物是否发生及得到，并协作解决实验遇到的问题并完成实验内容。待学生初步判定已得到最终产物，并得到指导教师认可后，方可结束实验操作。

学生提交最终化合物样品 10mg 进行质谱及 $^{1}H-NMR$ 测试，并根据谱图判断实验结果，总结实验内容，完成实验报告。提交实验报告及实验心得（纸板及电子版），并提交实验内容的 ppt 电子版。提交目标化合物样品用于今后药物分析开放实验的质量分析及药理学实验活性测试，完成学校规定的一系列开放实验的内容。

在实验结束一周内，全班同学以 ppt 讲解方式汇报工作，指导教师给予提问及点评，并对本次实验总结，批改报告后给予实验成绩。

【讨论题】

1. 你设计的化合物的设计目的及理论基础是什么，你设计的化合物属于哪类肾上腺素 β 受体阻断剂？

2. 你在实验中遇到哪些具体困难，是如何解决的？

3. 根据现有知识，如何判断所合成的目标化合物结构正确与否？

Ⅰ. Research of the design and synthesis of β-adrenergic receptor antagonist

Purpose

1. To design the structure and the synthetic route of a new β-adrenergic receptor antagonist independently so as to complete the synthesis and identification of the target compound.

2. To cultivate students' experimental skills, as well as their analytical skills, let students perform the experimental procedure on their own within the time required (64 classes) and experience the connotation and charm of scientific research.

3. To cultivate students' team spirit in the experiment.

Principle

Based on the structure-activity relationship of β-adrenergic receptor antagonist and the existing drugs, students are asked to design a new β-adrenergic receptor antagonist, both its structure and a reasonable synthetic route are required. Later complete the synthesis and identification of the target compound using their design.

Apparatus

Mechanical stirrer, magnetic stirrer, rotary evaporators (with cryogenic liquid cycle NG), low-temperature bath (−30℃), Autoclave, UV detector, high performance liquid chromatograph and general glass equipment.

Methods

All-day open.

Credit Hours

64 classes.

Procedure

1. Students are asked to design a new β-adrenergic receptor antagonist independently based on their knowledge of the structure-activity relationship of such compounds learned in class.

2. Search for the synthesis route based on the structure of the target compound using CAS SciFinder or Tomson integrity database and download the original literature from the databases such as Elsevier, CAS and CNKI, design the synthesis route of the target compound referring to routes of its analogues. It is better to keep the route no more than 6 steps. Also, students should determine the experiment condition of each step of reaction.

3. Submit a preliminary feasibility report to teachers at least 4 weeks before the experiment and explore the rationality of the target compound and the feasibility of the designed route with teachers.

4. After determining a reasonable synthetic route, each student should submit a manifest

which includes chemical materials, reagents and equipment required to the experiment center for preparation.

5. Each experiment group which consists 3 to 4 students should complete the experiment within the time required (64 classes), during which, students should identify whether the target compound or intermediate have been obtained in each step using thin-layer chromatography and UV analysis. Students are also asked to solve problems in cooperation and eventually finish the experiment.

6. The experiment can be considered finished after the teacher has confirmed the target compound has been reached and approved for ending the experiment.

7. Submit a 10 mg sample of the final product for MS and ^{1}H-NMR tests. Based on the spectrograms, students should finish experiment reports after analyzing the result and summarizing the experiment content.

8. Submit thc cxpcrimcnt rcport, experimental experience report (bothhardcopy and electronic version), and an electronic copy of experiment content in the form of ppt.

9. Submit a sample of the target compound for subsequent quality analysis and pharmacological activity tests.

10. All students should report work in the form of ppt presentations within 1 week after the end of the experiment, teachers will give questions and comments, summarize the experiment, and grade reports.

Discussion Questions

1. On what theoretical basis did you design your β-adrenergic receptor antagonist, and to which category should it be assorted?

2. What kind of problem have you encountered during the experiment? How did you solve it?

3. How to determine the compound you obtained to be the anticipated one based on the knowledge you have learned in class.

二、二氢吡啶类钙离子拮抗剂的设计合成、活性评价与杂质对产品质量的影响研究

【实验目的】

1. 使学生根据二氢吡啶类钙离子拮抗剂的构效关系，独立设计一条二氢吡啶类钙离子拮抗剂合理的合成路线，完成目标化合物的合成和质量分析等工作。

2. 使学生注重副产物的存在，了解如何解决在药物制备中副产物的产生和消除的问题，以保证质量。

3. 加深学生对药物杂质产生规律的认识，注重培养与设计药物具有类似结构杂质的消除和防止产生的科学思维方法，为以后的科研创新奠定基础。

【实验原理】

根据药物的构效关系，设计一条新的可行的二氢吡啶类钙离子拮抗剂合成路线，

并解决在药物制备中副产物的产生和消除的问题。

【仪器设备】

电动搅拌机、电磁搅拌机、旋转蒸发仪（附有低温液体循环仪）、低温浴槽（-30℃）、高压釜、紫外检测器、高效液相和常规玻璃仪器。

【实验方式】

全天候开放式。

【实验学时】

64 学时。

【实验内容】

1. 根据已学的二氢吡啶类钙离子拮抗剂的构效关系，运用药物设计的基本原理，自行设计二氢吡啶类钙离子拮抗剂的结构。

2. 根据设计的目标化合物结构，通过 CAS Scifinder 数据库及 Tomson integrity 数据库检索目标化合物的合成路线或类似物的合成路线，独立设计一合理可行的合成路线，并初步确定每步操作的适宜的实验条件，以减少或者消除副产物。

3. 实验开始 4 周前，要提交可行性实验报告，并与指导教师探讨目标化合物的合理性及设计路线的可行性以及杂质对产品质量的影响。

4. 确定一条合理可行的合成路线，提交实验内容需要的化学原料、试剂及仪器清单。由实验中心完成前期准备工作。

5. 学生以 3~4 人组成实验组，在规定时间内（一般 64 学时）独立完成实验内容。实验过程中，学生应通过薄层紫外鉴定等常规分析手段判断各步反应中间体及目标产物是否发生及得到，并协作解决实验遇到的问题完成实验内容。

6. 待学生初步判定已得到最终产物，并得到指导教师认可后，后方可结束实验操作。

7. 学生提交最终化合物样品 10mg 进行质谱及 $^{1}H-NMR$ 测试，并根据谱图判断实验结果，总结实验内容，完成实验报告。

8. 提交实验报告及实验心得（纸板及电子版），并提交实验内容的 ppt 电子版。

9. 提交目标化合物样品用于今后药物分析开放实验的质量分析及药理学实验活性测试，完成学校规定的一系列开放实验的内容。

10. 在实验结束一周内，全班同学以 ppt 讲解方式汇报工作，指导教师给予提问及点评，并对本次实验总结，批改报告后给予实验成绩。

【思考题】

1. 你设计的化合物的设计目的及理论基础是什么？

2. 在你设计的化合物合成过程中，会产生什么副产物，用什么方法可以减少或消除？

Ⅱ. Study of design, synthesis, activity evaluation and impurities impact on product quality of dihydropyridine calcium antagonists

Purpose

1. Design a reasonable synthetic route of a dihydropyridine calcium antagonist independently according to the structure-activity relationship, so as to complete the synthesis and quality analysis of target compounds.

2. To focus students' attention on by-products and to introduce them to solve problems regarding to the generation and elimination of impurities during the experiment and further assure the product quality.

3. To deepen students' cognition in the pattern of impurity generation, as well as their scientific thinking methods in the elimination or the avoidance of impurities akin to the designed drug, in which way, would establish a solid foundation for their future scientific research innovation.

Principle

Design a reasonable synthetic route of a dihydropyridine calcium antagonist independently according to the structure-activity relationship, and solve problems regarding to the avoidance and elimination of impurities during the experiment

Apparatus

Mechanical stirrer, magnetic stirrer, rotary evaporators (with cryogenic liquid cycle NG), low-temperature bath (−30℃), autoclave, UV detector, high performance liquid chromatograph and general glass equipment.

Methods

All-day open.

Credit Hours

64 classes.

Procedure

1. According to the relationship of structure and activity of dihydropyridine calcium antagonist learned in class and the basic principles of drug designing, students are asked to design the structure of a new dihydropyridine calcium antagonist.

2. Search for the synthetic route of the target compounds according its structure from the CAS SciFinder database and the Tomson integrity database, design a reasonable and achievable synthetic route independently. Also, students are asked to determine the appropriate experiment conditions of each step for impurity elimination.

3. Submit a preliminary feasibility report to teachers at least 4 weeks before the experiment and explore the rationality of the target compound and the feasibility of the designed route with teachers.

4. After determining a reasonable synthetic route, submit a manifest including chemical materials, reagents and equipment required to the experiment center for preparation.

5. Each experiment group which consists 3 to 4 students should complete the experiment within the time required(64 classes). During which, students should identify whether the target compound or intermediate have been obtained in each step using thin-layer chromatography and UV analysis. Students are also asked to solve problems in cooperation and eventually finish the experiment.

6. The experiment can be considered finished after the teacher has confirmed the target compound has been reached and approved for ending the experiment.

7. Submit a 10 mg sample of the final product for MS and ^{1}H-NMR tests. Based on the spectrograms, students should finish experiment reports after analyzing the result and summarizing the experiment content.

8. Submit the experiment report, experimental experience report (both hardcopy and electronic version), and an electronic copy of experiment content in the form of ppt.

9. Submit a sample of the target compound for subsequent quality analysis and pharmacological activity tests.

10. All students should report work in the form of ppt presentations within 1 week after the end of the experiment, teachers will give questions and comments, summarize the experiment, and grade reports.

Questions

1. What is the purpose of your design and what is its theoretical basis?

2. During the synthesis of your designed compound, what by-products would it create? What is the way to diminish or eliminate such impurities?

三、尿嘧啶衍生物的抗代谢物的设计与生物活性测定及体内分析

【实验目的】

1. 加深学生对体内活性物质的深度认识，运用药物设计的基本理论，进行创新性研究。

2. 培养学生对非本专业的科学研究成果的消化和吸收能力。

3. 利用最新科学研究结果的创新能力和科学研究的团队精神。

【实验原理】

以现有的抗代谢药物设计原理以及尿嘧啶抗肿瘤药物的知识为基础，完成尿嘧啶衍生物的抗代谢物的设计及生物活性评价。

【仪器设备】

电动搅拌机、电磁搅拌机、旋转蒸发仪（附有低温液体循环仪）、低温浴槽（－30℃）、高压釜、紫外检测器、高效液相和常规玻璃仪器。

【实验方式】

全天候开放式。

【实验学时】

64 学时。

【实验内容】

1. 归纳总结现有的抗代谢药物设计原理以及尿嘧啶抗肿瘤药物的知识，独立设计一个尿嘧啶衍生物的抗代谢药物。

2. 根据设计的目标化合物结构，从学校现有的 Elsevier、CAS、CNKI 及中国知网等数据库资源下载原始文献，参考同类药物的合成路线，设计目标化合物的合成路线。

3. 实验开始 4 周前，要提交可行性实验报告，并与指导教师探讨目标化合物的合理性及设计路线的可行性。

4. 确定一条合理可行的合成路线，提交实验内容需要的化学原料、试剂及仪器清单。由实验中心完成前期准备工作。

5. 学生以 3 ~4 人组成实验组，在规定时间内（一般 64 学时）独立完成实验内容。实验过程中，学生应通过薄层紫外鉴定等常规分析手段判断各步反应中间体及目标产物是否发生及得到，并协作解决实验遇到的问题并完成实验内容。

6. 待学生初步判定已得到最终产物，并得到指导教师认可后，后方可结束实验操作。

7. 学生提交最终化合物样品 10mg 进行质谱及 ^{1}H-NMR 测试，并根据谱图判断实验结果，总结实验内容，完成实验报告。

8. 提交实验报告及实验心得（纸板及电子版），并提交实验内容的 ppt 电子版。

9. 提交目标化合物样品用于今后药物分析开放实验的质量分析及药理学实验活性测试，完成学校规定的一系列开放实验的内容。

10. 在实验结束一周内，全班同学以 ppt 讲解方式汇报工作，指导教师给予提问及点评，并对本次实验总结，批改报告后给予实验成绩。

【思考题】

1. 你设计的化合物的设计作用机制和构效关系是什么？是否比其他尿嘧啶衍生物的抗代谢物有优势，优势是什么？

2. 你在实验中遇到哪些问题，是如何解决的？

3. 总结一下你感觉在实验过程中需要注意的事项？

Ⅲ. Design, bioassay and analysis *in vivo* of Uracil derivatives anti-metabolites

Purpose

1. To deepen students' understanding of activity material in vivo. Use the basic theories of drug designing to conduct innovative research.

2. To train students of the digestion and absorption capacity of the research results beyond the field of profession.

3. To cultivate students' innovative capability using the latest scientific findings, also team spirit during scientific research.

Principle

Based on the existing designing principles of anti-metabolites and the knowledge of uracil antitumor drugs, finish the design and biological activity evaluation of uracil derivatives anti-metabolites.

Equipment

Mechanical stirrer, magnetic stirrer, rotary evaporators (with cryogenic liquid cycle NG), low-temperature bath (−30℃), autoclave, UV detector, high performance liquid chromatograph and general glass equipment.

Methods

All-day open.

Credit Hours

64classes.

Procedure

1. Summarize the existing design principles of anti-metabolites and the knowledge of uracil antitumor drugs and design a new uracil derivatives anti-metabolite independently.

2. Download the original literature from Elsevier、CAS、CNKI database based on the structure of the designed target compound, design the synthetic route of the target compound referring to routes of its analogues.

3. Submit a preliminary feasibility report 4 weeks before the experiment begins and discuss the rationality of the target compound and the feasibility of the designed route with tutors.

4. After determining a reasonable synthetic route, each student should submit a manifest which includes chemical materials, reagents and equipment required in the experiment to the experiment center for preparation.

5. Each experiment group which consists 3 to 4 students should complete the experiment within the time required (64 classes). During which, students should identify whether the target compound or intermediate have been obtained in each step using thin－layer chromatography and UV analysis. Students are also asked to solve problems in cooperation and eventually finish the experiment.

6. The experiment can be considered finished after the teacher has confirmed the target compound has been reached and approved for ending the experiment.

7. Submit a 10 mg sample of the final compound for the MS and ^{1}H-NMR tests. Based on the spectrograms, students should finish experiment report after analyzing the result and summarizing the experiment content.

8. Submit the experiment report, experimental experience report (both hardcopy and e-

lectronic version), and an electronic copy of experiment content in the form of ppt.

9. Submit a sample of the target compound for subsequent quality analysis and pharmacological activity tests.

10. All students should report work in the form of ppt presentations within 1 week after the end of the experiment, teachers will give questions and comments, summarize the experiment, and grade reports.

Questions

1. What are the mechanism and structure-activity relationships of the compound you designed? What is its advantage over other uracil derivatives anti-metabolites, if any?

2. What kind of problems have you encountered during the experiment? How did you solve it?

3. Summarize the matters that you think should be paid attention to during the experiment.

四、前体药物的设计与评价（抗癌、抗菌、糖代谢皮质激素、非甾体抗炎药物）

【实验目的】

1. 加深学生对药物体内代谢的认识。
2. 培养学生独立设计一个前体药物，并设计一条合理可行的合成路线。
3. 培养学生的药化实验技能及再创新能力。

【实验原理】

依据课堂上掌握的前体药物的知识，设计一前体药物，并为这一前体药物寻找一条合理可行的合成路线。

【仪器设备】

电动搅拌机、电磁搅拌机、旋转蒸发仪（附有低温液体循环仪）、低温浴槽（-30℃）、高压釜、紫外检测器、高效液相和常规玻璃仪器。

【实验方式】

全天候开放式。

【实验学时】

64 学时。

【实验内容】

1. 归纳总结现有的前体药物的有关知识，并根据这些知识设计一个前体药物。

2. 根据设计的目标化合物，通过 CAS Scifinder 数据库及 Tomson integrity 数据库检索目标化合物的合成路线或类似物的合成路线，独立设计一合理可行的合成路线，并初步确定每步操作的实验条件。

3. 实验开始 4 周前，要提交可行性实验报告，并与指导教师探讨目标化合物的合理性及设计路线的可行性。

4. 确定一条合理可行的合成路线，提交实验内容需要的化学原料、试剂及仪器清单。由实验中心完成前期准备工作。

5. 学生以3～4人组成实验组，在规定时间内（一般64学时）独立完成实验内容。实验过程中，学生应通过薄层紫外鉴定等常规分析手段判断各步反应中间体及目标产物是否发生及得到，并协作解决实验遇到的问题并完成实验内容。

6. 待学生初步判定已得到最终产物，并得到指导教师认可后，后方可结束实验操作。

7. 学生提交最终化合物样品10mg进行质谱及^{1}H－NMR测试，并根据谱图判断实验结果，总结实验内容，完成实验报告。

8. 提交实验报告及实验心得（纸板及电子版），并提交实验内容的ppt电子版。

9. 提交目标化合物样品用于今后药物分析开放实验的质量分析及药理学实验活性测试，完成学校规定的一系列开放实验的内容。

10. 在实验结束一周内，全班同学以ppt讲解方式汇报工作，指导教师给予提问及点评，并对本次实验总结，批改报告后给予实验成绩。

【思考题】

1. 什么叫前体药物，前体药物的主要来源有那些？
2. 你设计的前体药物是通过什么途径设计的？
3. 你在实验中遇到哪些问题，是如何解决的？

Ⅳ. Design and evaluation of prodrugs（anti-cancer，anti-bacterial，glucose metabolism cortical hormones，non-steroidal anti-inflammatory drugs）

Purpose

1. To deepen students' understanding of drug metabolism *in vivo*.

2. To train students to design a prodrug independently as well as a reasonable and achievable synthetic route.

3. To cultivate students' medicinal chemistry experimental skills and re－innovation ability.

Principle

Design a prodrug and find a reasonable and achievable synthetic route for the prodrug based on the knowledge learned in class.

Equipment

Mechanical stirrer，magnetic stirrer，rotary evaporators（with cryogenic liquid cycle NG），low-temperature bath（－30℃），autoclave，UV detector，high performance liquid chromatograph and general glass equipment.

Methods

All-day open.

Credit Hours

64 classes.

Procedure

1. Design a prodrug based on the existing knowledge of the prodrug.

2. Search for the synthetic route of the target compounds according its structure from the CAS SciFinder database and the Tomson integrity database, design a reasonable and achievable synthetic route independently and determine the experimental conditions of each step of reaction preliminarily.

3. Submit a feasibility report 4 weeks before the experiment begins and discuss the rationality of the target compounds and the feasibility of the designed route with tutors.

4. Determine a reasonable and achievable synthetic route, submit a manifest of chemical materials, reagents and equipments that is needed in the experiment to experiment center for preparation work.

5. Form experimental group with 3-4 persons and finish the experimental items independently within the required period of time (64 classes). During which, students should identify whether the target compound have been obtained in each step using thin – layer chromatography and UV analysis. Students are also asked to solve problems in cooperation and eventually finish the experiment.

6. The experiment can be considered finished after the teacher has confirmed the target compound has been reached and approved for ending the experiment.

7. Submit a 10 mg sample of the final compound for the MS and ^1H – NMR tests. Based on the spectrograms, students should finish experiment reports after analyzing the result and summarizing the experiment content.

8. Submit the experiment report, experimental experience report (both hardcopy and electronic version), and an electronic copy of experiment content in the form of ppt.

9. Submit a sample of the target compound for subsequent quality analysis and pharmacological activity tests.

10. All students should report work in the form of ppt presentations within 1 week after the end of the experiment, teachers will give questions and comments, summarize the experiment, and grade reports.

Questions

1. What is prodrug, and what is the main source of prodrugs?

2. Through what pathway did you designed your prodrug?

3. What are the problems youhave encountered in the experiment? How did you solve it?

附录　重要的实验方法

一、液体化合物的分离与提纯方法

有机合成产生的液体化合物其分离纯化一般采用蒸馏的方法。根据待分离组分和理化性性质的不同，蒸馏可以分为简单蒸馏和精馏（分馏）；根据装置系统内的压力不同又可分为常压和减压蒸馏。对于沸点差极小的组分分离或对产物纯度要求极高的分离，则可应用高真空技术。参见《有机化学实验》。

二、固体化合物的提纯方法

化学合成药物的纯度和质量是关系到人身安危的重大问题。为了获得高纯度的药品，对最终成品及关键中间体必须进行提纯和精制。固体物质一般采用结晶（重结晶、分级结晶等）或升华的方法进行纯化。参见《有机化学实验》。

三、常用色谱方法

色谱（又称层析）是一种物理的分离方法。它的分离原理是使混合物中各组分在两相间进行分配，其中一相是不动的，称为固定相，另一相是携带混合物流过此固定相的流体，称为流动相。当流动相中所含混合物经过固定相时，就会与固定相发生作用。由于各组分在性质和结构上有差异，与固定相发生作用的大小、强弱也有差异，因此在同一推动力作用下，不同组分在固定相中的滞留时间有长有短，从而按先后不同的次序从固定相中流出。这种借助在两相间分配差异而使混合物中各组分分离的技术，称为色谱法。

（一）薄层色谱

薄层色谱（TLC）是一种简单实用的实验技术，属固液层析。

一般薄层色谱的固定相是硅胶或氧化铝，属吸附层析。在层析过程中，吸附剂对样品中各组分的吸附力不同，当展开剂流过时，各组分被展开剂从吸附剂上解析下来的难易程度不同，从而造成各组分移动时的速度差别，而达到分离的目的。

薄层色谱可以用来分离混合物、鉴定精制化合物、测量混合物中各组分的含量、测定样品纯度。其展开时间短，几十分钟就能达到分离目的，分离效率高，还可用制备板分离几毫克到几百毫克的样品。在药物合成实验中，还常用来跟踪反应进程和确定反应的终点。薄层色谱特别适用于挥发性小的化合物以及在高温下化学性质不稳定的化合物的分析。

（二）柱色谱

柱色谱是通过层析柱来实现分离的，主要用于大量化合物的分离。层析柱内装有固体吸附剂，也就是固定相，如氧化铝或硅胶等。液体样品从柱顶加入，在柱的顶部被吸附剂吸附，然后从柱的顶部加入有机溶剂也就是展开剂进行洗脱。由于吸附剂对各组分的吸附能力不同，各组分以不同速度下移，被吸附较弱的组分在流动相里的含量较高，以较快的速度下移。各组分随溶剂按一定顺序从层析柱下端流处，分段收集流出液，再用薄层色谱来鉴定各组分。

柱色谱的分离条件可以套用该样品的薄层色谱条件，分离效果亦相同。

（三）纸色谱

纸色谱是以滤纸为载体，用一定的溶剂系统展开而达到分离、分析目的的色谱方法。此法可用于定性，亦可用于分离制备微量样品。纸色谱的原理是分配色谱。滤纸是载体，水为固定相，展开剂为流动相。试样在固定相水与流动相展开剂之间连续抽提，依靠溶质在两相间的分配系数不同而达到分离的目的。物质在两相之间有固定的分配系数，在纸色谱上也有固定的比移值。

纸色谱法的一般操作时，将待试样品溶于适当溶剂，点样于滤纸一端，另用适当挑选的溶剂系统，从点样的一端通过毛细现象向另一端展开。展开完毕，滤纸取出阴干，以适当显色剂显色，即得纸层析色谱。样品层析往往用比移值 R_f 来表示某一化合物在纸色谱中的位置。

（四）高效液相色谱

高效液相色谱（HPLC）是一种具有高灵敏度、高选择性的高效、快速分离分析技术，广泛应用于医药分析的各个领域。在药品质量控制如主要成分的定性定量分析、杂质的限量检查和测定、稳定性考察等、药物合成反应的监测、药物体内过程和代谢动力学研究、中药的成分研究及人体内源活性物质的测定中，HPLC 都是重要的分析手段。

例如，β-肾上腺素受体拮抗剂类药物均为手性分子的外消旋体，其对映异构体的药效学差异显著。近年来在这些药物的对映体选择性 HPLC 分析方法研究上取得了令人瞩目的进展。常见的 HPLC 手性拆分方法有手性固定相直接拆分法、手性试剂衍生化法和手性流动相添加法。

例如，采用柱前衍生化测定普萘洛尔对映体：

1. 色谱条件

色谱柱：Micro Pak SP　C8 柱（15 mm × 14 mm）

流动相：醋酸钠（0.02 mol / L，pH 4.0）-乙腈（30 : 70）

流速：2 ml / min

检测：荧光，265 nm / 345nm。

2. 样品测定　样品经硼酸－磷酸二氢钠缓冲液（0.10 mol / L，pH 用氢氧化钠调至 8.5）稀释，混合后取样品溶液 20μl，加入（+）-1-(9-芴基)-乙基甲酰氯（FLEC）衍生化试剂 20μl，反应 10 min 后，取 10μl 进样。保留时间：（－）-普萘洛尔衍生物为 6.549 min；（+）－普萘洛尔衍生物为 7.070 min；FLEC 为 12.1 min。

四、光学异构药物的拆分

药物的立体结构与生物活性密切相关。含手性中心的药物，其对映体之间的生物活性往往有很大的差异。研究表明药物立体异构体药效差异的主要原因是他们与受体结合的差异。

近年来人们对光学异构体间的药效有了长足的认识，以单一异构体供药用已引起各方面的重视，今后的新药研制将日益朝着单一对应体药物的方向发展。

对应异构体的药物一般可以通过不对称合成或拆分方法得到。然而就目前医药工业生产而言，尚未有成熟的不对称合成方法用于药物的大量生产，因此，拆分仍然是获得手性药物的重要方法。常用的光学异构药物的拆分方法与拆分原理包括：

（一）播种结晶法

在外消旋体的饱和溶液中加入其中一种纯的单一光学异构体（左旋或右旋）结晶，使溶液对这种异构体成过饱和状态，然后在一定温度下该过饱和的旋光异构体优先大量析出结晶，迅速过滤得到单一光学异构体。再往滤液中加入一定量的消旋体，则溶液中另一种异构体达到饱和，经冷却过滤后得到另一个单一光学异构体，经过如此反复操作，连续拆分便可以交叉获得左旋体和右旋体。

播种结晶法的优点是不需用光学拆分剂，因此原料消耗少、成本低。而且该法操作较简单、所需设备少、生产周期短、母液可套用多次、拆分收率高。但该法仅适用于两种对映体晶体独立存在的外消旋混合物的拆分，对大部分只含一个手性碳原子的互为对映体的光学异构药物，无法用播种结晶法进行拆分。另外，播种结晶法拆分的条件控制也较麻烦，制备过饱和溶液的温度和冷却析晶的温度都必须通过实验加以确定，拆分所得的光学异构体的光学纯度不高。

（二）形成非对映异构盐法

对映异构体一般都具有相同的理化性质，用重结晶、分馏、萃取及常规色谱法不能分离。而非对映异构体的理化性质有一定差异，因此利用消旋体的化学性质，使其与某一光学活性化合物（即拆分剂）作用生成两种非对映异构盐，再利用它们的物理性质（如溶解度）不同，将他们分离，最后除去拆分剂，便可以得到光学纯的异构体。目前国内外大部分光学活性药物，均用此法生产。

（三）酶拆分法

利用酶对光学活性异构体选择性的酶解作用，使外消旋体中的一个光学异构体优先酶解，而另一个难酶解，后者被保留而达到分离的目的。

（四）色谱拆分法

利用气相和液相色谱可以测定光学异构体纯度，进行实验室少量样品制备，推断光学异构体的构型和构象等。

Appendix　Important empirical methods

1. Separation and purification of liquid compounds

The principal method chosen for the separation and purification of liquid compounds in organic synthesis is distillation. According to the difference of the physical and chemical properties of the substance concerned, distillation may be divided into simple distillation and rectification (fractional distillation); and could also be divided into atmospheric distillation and reduced-pressure distillation depending on the difference of the pressure in the system. If the boiling-points of the liquid components are close together or the products need high purity, high vacuum technology is required.

2. Purification of solid compounds

The purity and quality of chemical synthesis drugs are an important problem to the security of human beings. Important intermediates and final products must be purified and refined to get high purity drugs. Crystallization (recrystallization, the fractionation crystallization) is probably the most frequently used method in purifying organic solids. See *experiment of organic chemstry*.

3. Chromatography

Chromatography (also called laminar analysis) is a physical separate method. The separate principle is that the components of mixtures are distributed to two phases, one of the phases is immobility is called stationary phase and the other phase taking along the mixtures to move along the stationary phase is called moving phase. When the mixtures in the moving phase move along the stationary phase, they react with stationary phase. Because of different properties and structures among components, they also have different force reacting with stationary phase, so the retention time of different components in the stationary phase under the identical driving force is different, and the components elute from stationary phase with different sequence. The technology depending on the distributed difference between two phases makes each component of the mixtures separated is called chromatography.

(1) Thin-layer chromatography

Thin-layer chromatography is a simple and useful empirical technology, it belongs to liquid-solid chromatography.

In generally, the stationary phase of thin-layer chromatography is silica gel or alumina, it belongs to absorption laminar analysis. In the process of laminar analysis, the absorbent has different absorbing ability with each component, when the eluting solvent moves, each component resolving from absorbent has different speed, and that makes each component remove in different speed to achieve separation.

Thin-layer chromatography may be used to separate mixtures, identify and refine compounds, measure the contents of component and the purity of sample in each mixture. The eluting time is short, and it takes several ten minutes to achieve separation with high efficiency of this method, and it could also separate few mg to hundred mg sample product with prepared layer. In the experiment of drug synthesis, it is always used to track the process of the reaction and make sure the ending of the reaction. Thin-layer chromatography is especially fit for analyzing the compounds with little volatility or instablility under high temperature .

(2) Column Chromatography

Column chromatography completes separation by chromatographic column; it is chiefly used for separating massive compounds. Chromatographic column loads powdered solid such as alumina or silica gel which is also called stationary phase. A solution of the mixture is then poured into the top of the column and passed slowly down the tube by adding further sample of the eluting solvent. The components in the mixture are separated as they move down the column, according to their relative strengths of absorption by the stationary phase. Each composition has different speed in removing. The compositions which are absorbed weakly have high content in the moving phase and remove with fast speed. The solution of the separated components may be collected as they are eluted from the bottom of the chromatographic column in certain sequence, and each component can be identified with thin - layer chromato - graphy.

The separation condition of column chromatography may adopt similarly condition of thin - layer chromatography, and the effect of separation is identical.

(3) Paper chromatography

Paper chromatography is based on filter paper as carrier, by certain solvent system developing to achieve separation and analysis. The method could be used for qualitation, and could also be used for separating and preparing slight sample. The principle of it is partition chromatography. The filter paper is carrier, water is stationary phase and eluting solvent is moving phase. Sample relying on the difference of partition coefficient of the solutes extract continuously between the stationary phase and the moving phase to achieve separation. The components have fixed partition coefficient between the two phases, and they also have fixed rate of flow (R_f) value on the Paper Chromatography.

Generally operate the paper chromatography, the sample is dissolved in suitable solvent, and a drop of the solution of the mixture is applied on the line, the suitable moving solvent system chosen gradually moves up the paper by capillary action the component of the mixture. After the development, the filter paper is brought out and dried in the shad, with certain chromogenic agent to show color to get Paper Chromatography. In laminar analysis of the sample, rate of flow (R_f) value is used to demonstrate the position of the spots of certain compound in the paper Chromatography.

(4) High Performance Liquid Chromatography

High Performance Liquid Chromatography (HPLC) is to have high sensitivity, high selectivity, high efficiency, quick separation and analysis technology, and generally is applied in every field of the medicine analysis. To control the quality of drug such as the qualitation and quantitation of the major compositions, the limited examination and determination of impurity, the investigation of stability, the monitoring of the reaction for drug synthesis, the research on the drug in internal process, the research on drug in metabolism and kinesics, the research on the compositions of traditional Chinese drug and the determination of endogenous compositions of human, HPLC is an important analytic method.

For example, the drugs of β-adrenergic antagonists are all racemic bodies as chiral molecules, the difference of those enantiomers in pharmacodynamics is very distinguished. In recent years, the research on the selectivity of these drugs' racemic bodies by HPLC analytic method has achieved remarkable development. General methods of the chiral separation in HPLC are direct resolution, derivatization of chiral reagents and the addition of chiral moving phase.

For example, derivatization before column to determine the enantiomer of propranolol:

a. the condition of color spectrum:

Chromatographic column: Micro Pak SP C8 column (15mm × 14mm)

Moving phase: sodium acetate (0.02mol/l, pH 4.0)-methyl cyanide (30 : 70)

Flow rate: 2ml/min

Determination: fluorescence 265nm/345nm.

b. determining sample : the sample dilute with boric acid-sodium dihydrogen phosphate balance solution (0.10mol/L, sodium hydroxide adjust to pH 8.5) . After that take the solution of simple products 20μl, add to the derivatization of (+)-1-(9-fluorene)-ethyl formyl chloride(FLEC) 20μl, after reacting for 10 min, bring 10μl to inject. Retention time: the derivatization of (−)-propranolol is 6.549min; the derivatization of (+)-propranolol is 7.070min; and the FLEC is 12.1min.

4. The resolution of optical isomerism drugs

The stereochemical structure of the drugs has compacted relationship to the bioactivity. The enantiomers of the drugs containing chiral center often have largely different bioactivity. The research shows that the primary reason that the drug action difference of stereoisomer is the difference in integrating with the receptors.

In recent years, people have adequate knowledge of the drugs action among optical isomers, and prescribe drugs with single enanotiomer has brought out great attention in all parts; nowadays the development of new drugs will face the development of the single enanotiomer trend.

In generally, the drugs with enanotiomer may be obtained by applying the asymmetric synthesis and resolution. However, as far as the product of the medicinal industry, there are not ripe methods of asymmetric synthesis to apply large scale drugs produce; therefore resolution is still the important method to gain chiral drugs. The general method and principle of resolution about optical isomers include:

(1) Seed crystallization

One of the pure and single optical isomer in the racemic body is being joined into the saturated solution of it, and the isomer in the solution shows the condition of supersaturation, then in certain temperature, firstly the racemic body in the solution of the supersaturation educes massive crystal, and the solution is being filtered to get single optical isomer. Then certain racemic is being added into colatus solution, and the other isomer in the solution achieve saturation, then the solution is being cooled and filtered to gain the other single optical isomer, by such repetatus operation and continuous resolution, we may get single L – isomer and R – isomer.

The merit of the seed crystallization is that there is no need of optical resolution agent, so it consumes small raw materials and the cost of it is low. And this method has simple operation, small equipment needing, short cycle for production, many times using the mother liquor, high yield of resolution. But the method only could apply two crystals of enantiomer which exist without the other, and the drugs containing optical isomer which just contain one chiral carbon could not carry out resolution with seed crystallization. In addition, the control condition of the seed crystallization resolution is very trouble, and the temperature in which prepared the supersaturated solution and cooled to educe crystal must need the experiment to be ascertained, so the optical purity of optical isomer which gets from resolution is not high.

(2) Form the salt of diastereoisomer

Enantiomer generally has identical physico – chemical property, and could not be separated by recrystallization, distillation, extraction and routine chromatography. But the physico – chemical property of diastereoisomer is different, so we could apply the chemical property of racemic acting with some optical activity compound (also called resolution agent) to product two kinds of salt of diastereoisomer which can be separated by the difference of physical property of them (such as solubility), eventually the resolution agent is removed to get the optical pure isomer. At present, the major optical activity drugs are prepared by this method at home and abroad.

(3) The resolution of enzymes catalysis

Enzymes has selective enzymolysis to the optical activity isomer, which make one optical isomer of racemic body degrades, the other is hard to degrade, then to achieve separation.

(4) Chromatography resolution

Preparing slight sample and concluding the configuration and conformation of the optical isomer apply that Gas Chromatogram and Liquid Chromatogram which can determine the purity of the optical isomer.